Something Understood

Reflections on Discipleship and Disability

by
Graham Evans

Grosvenor House
Publishing Limited

This book is published by
Grosvenor House Publishing Ltd
28-30 High Street, Guildford, Surrey, GU1 3EL.
www.grosvenorhousepublishing.co.uk

The Scripture quotations contained herein are from The New Revised
Standard version of the Bible, Anglicised edition, copyright 1989, 1995
by the Division of Christian Education of the National Council of the
Churches of Christ in the United States of America and are used
by permission. All rights reserved.

A CIP record for this book
is available from the British Library

ISBN 978-1-78148-975-8

For Dad

He would have been surprised by quite a few things in these pages but his faith and political convictions helped launch me on the Christian journey.

Alan Ffoulkes Evans
(1923 - 2013)

I Way Markers
2

II Down South
10

III Out West
24

IV Downtown
40

V Back East
54

VI Up North
70

VII Travelling Companions
84

VIII Blue Highways
94

IX Homeward Bound?
106

1

I
Way Markers

One June afternoon in 1992 I stood on the cliffs of eastern England looking down on Robin Hood's Bay. It was one of the most satisfying moments of my life. My brother and I had just completed a fortnight walking across northern England through the Lake District and the Yorkshire Dales and across the North Yorks Moors. This coast-to-coast walk is not a designated long-distance path but was devised by the eccentric genius and doyen of walkers Alfred Wainwright. He himself felt that it was a much superior walk than some of the more "official" long-distance treks such as the Pennine Way. Certainly a walk could not have a more clearly defined beginning and end. You dip your boots into the Irish Sea and a fortnight or so later, accidents and blisters permitting, you do the same in the North Sea. In the twenty years and more since I did the walk it has become increasingly popular. Careful minor adjustments have been made to the suggested route. Coast-to-coast signposts abound (and there is even a coast-to-coast fish and chip shop). It must be almost impossible to lose your way on such a well-defined and publicised route.

Much of which feels like a helpful metaphor for how I viewed the Christian journey in my earlier years. It had a defined beginning. Not with my infant baptism but with my response as a teenager to the call to accept Jesus as my personal saviour and welcome him into my heart. It would have a defined ending when, as one of the saved, I would after death, to use the Salvation Army phrase, be "promoted to glory." And in between a clearly defined set of doctrines had been provided to keep me on the narrow way. These had been clearly set out in the Scriptures which, properly interpreted, contained all things necessary for salvation. We rejoiced that, as the old chorus put it, we had been lifted from sinking sands, "from shades of night to planes of light."

What seems to be true now is that a rather different kind of path came increasingly to be a more accurate metaphor for my Christian journey. In Robert Macfarlane's book *The Old Ways* I came across a description of the ancient road The Icknield Way. This rises somewhere in southern Norfolk and runs west and south until eventually reaching Dorset. Its beginning and end are in doubt, it is no longer possible to trace its route in some parts, and indeed some question whether it was one pathway at all but see it as a series of parallel tracks. It has an "uncertain history, disputed route and debatable limits." (1)

This seems to resonate as an image with the Christian journey I have been on for quite a long time. Where the beginning and the ending are lost in mystery; where the Way is often difficult to discern; where there are far fewer if any dogmatic or ethical certainties. Rather a lot of the hymns I am invited to sing in Sunday worship I join in because they are part of my cultural inheritance rather than because I can relate to the lyrics. It's a little like the guilty pleasure to be found in listening to a performance of "Land of Hope and Glory" even though you are fully aware that the words are mainly nonsensical. I now find particular difficulty in relating to the language of sacrifice and atonement which was at the centre of the style of Christianity in which I grew up. Traditional Nonconformist worship no longer seems to be a means of grace for me on any but the most exceptional occasions. The gap between much of what happens in Sunday worship and my lived experience often appears more like a chasm.

Attempting to analyse how the journey has brought me to this point, some factors are deeply personal whilst others are the product of belonging to what many are calling a post-Christian society. Whether it is true or not that the Christian metanarrative as a whole has lost credibility, it is certainly the case that some traditional expressions of that no longer resonate with many people, including those who are attempting to reformulate Christian believing in ways that make sense to them. So for example we no longer find the Pilgrim's Progress understanding of the journey helpful. Life no longer feels like travelling through a variety of temptations and difficulties as a prelude to arriving at the celestial city. I notice that none of the hymns from the "Death, Judgement and Future Life" section of the *Methodist Hymn Book* (which was the standard Methodist collection until the 1980s) were included in its successors *Hymns and Psalms* and *Singing the Faith*. Christian focus nowadays seems to be concerned more with how we are making the journey itself rather than on what might be its destination. Not that the idea of pilgrimage in itself is defunct. A 2010 Festival of religious films had the title "Journeys of Faith Journeys of Hope" and encouraged the connection between pilgrimage as an inner search and journeying as a migration brought about by necessity. Even more recently, a bestselling novel of 2012 made extensive use of the theme of pilgrimage. (2) Harold Fry has no conventional religious belief but Christian motifs of faith, redemption and transformation are scattered throughout the story of his journey and in some ways he is a Christ-like figure. The epigraph for the novel is the first verse of John Bunyan's "Who would true valour see" but we are a long way removed from Christian making his way through temptations which might divert him from the narrow path of salvation.

For me, a further important factor has been the study of contemporary theological thinking. When I left home to study theology at university, one of the mentors of my teenage years said to me "Don't let them destroy your faith." In a sense he was right: immersion in theology meant that the faith of my earlier years was changed almost beyond recognition. But from

5

the outset I found that an exhilarating experience. Reading theology has sometimes been baffling, but more often liberating. Mind you, it took a while before the necessity of some discernment about new ideas became obvious to me. At first what were quite eccentric positions – such as the New Testament lecturer who told us that without doubt Lazarus was the author of the Fourth Gospel – were lapped up indiscriminately!

Exposure to theological thinking and very different understandings of Christian faith have been interwoven with personal experience which has necessitated facing a series of challenges. These have included (although the list is not exhaustive as they say!): the deep pain of some personal relationships, a crisis in my sense of vocation to ordained ministry, a lengthy period of wrestling with anxiety and depression, my part in a marriage which whilst it brought lots of happiness ended in failure, the onset of chronic disability with the concomitant necessity to accept early retirement. That reads like a very gloomy list when presented baldly like that! The broader intention is to see how such experiences might have interacted with Christian understanding on my journey – more about some of that later. It is certainly true that there have been lots of encounters with what Harry Williams called that tricky customer joy along the way as well. The journey has rarely had that feel of rather wearied ennui captured by Dickens:

"And thus ever, by day and night, under the sun and under the stars, climbing the dusty hills and toiling along the weary plains, journeying by land and journeying by sea, coming and going so strangely, to meet and to act and react on one another, move all we restless travellers through the pilgrimage of life." (3)

I recall a concert given by the Canadian singer Leonard Cohen. In between songs, he spoke honestly and with self-deprecating humour about his own struggles with depression. Over the years he had been prescribed a host of different antidepressants but "I had to give them all up because cheerfulness kept breaking in!" For me, the periods when cheerfulness failed to break in at all have been recurring but relatively infrequent. Nevertheless, one of my favourite surreal moments was provided by a volunteer steward at a noted tourist destination who welcomed me with the words "You people (that is to say people in wheelchairs) are always so cheerful." Interesting!

It may be that looking back on the journey from late middle age is partly prompted by a wistful nostalgia. Along the lines of, I wonder what happened to that girl who I really fancied but was too shy to approach. And what was her name? But perhaps there is more here than simply nostalgia. Being 60-ish could be a good time to look back and reflect on how decisions made, decisions imposed and seemingly random circumstances have shaped the direction and style of one's journey. Hopefully sufficient insight has been gained that the reflection doesn't simply become an exercise in donning rose tinted spectacles or practising self-justification.

At any rate, I have entitled these reflections *Something Understood*. The phrase is the last one in a remarkable poem entitled *Prayer (I)* by the 17th century priest and poet George Herbert. In it Herbert gives us a whole series of evocative phrases pointing to aspects of spiritual life. For me "something understood" is an enigmatic phrase. It suggests convictions that have been worked out or arrived at but also that much more is not understood. There is ambiguity, puzzlement, mystery about the journey of faith. I recall many years ago hearing a sermon by John Habgood, later to become Archbishop of York, around the theme "the more you know, the less you know you know." Something understood suggests a pilgrim who is both a believer and an agnostic, and that is where the journey to date has brought me. To describe these pages as "a spiritual memoir" sounds dreadfully pretentious but I guess it is something along those lines that I am attempting to produce.

It is, I suppose, a little ironic that I should be reflecting on journeys at a time in life when I am less mobile than I have been at any time since my earliest months on the planet. I have been a full-time wheelchair user for several years and will be for the rest of my life. Outings have to be planned with a great deal of care and almost always require the assistance of friends or my personal assistant. I spend more time than I ever have previously in my adult life at home. The undoubted link between walking (or horse riding in the case of John Wesley) and thinking is of no benefit to me. However, I am encouraged by reading that part of the Rule of St Benedict "is clear that alternative models of monastic life that are based on peripatetic wandering have a high risk of being corrupted. He has a name for monks of this sort – gyrovagues – who "spend their whole lives lodging in different regions and different monasteries three or four days at a time, always wandering and never stable." (4) Perhaps there is much to be said for being rooted in one place, and not just for those in a monastic community (it is not difficult to spot the gyrovague tendency in some 21st-century churchgoers!). The composer Vaughan Williams claimed that "Only a "local" or even "parochial" artist can become a "universal musician." He believed that "if the roots of your art are firmly planted in your own soil and that soil has anything to give you, you may still gain the whole world and not lose your own souls." (5) That is surely true of Christian discipleship as well as music.

So whilst as the old song has it, "I don't get around much anymore," the following pages will describe some journeys plucked from memory or imagination and use them as metaphors, starting points for some reflections on different aspects of the Christian journey which have come to seem important to me. The itinerary will take us down south, up north, out west and back east. In the hope that one person's journey might have some resonances for others as they travel.

(1) Robert Macfarlane: The Old Ways (Hamish Hamilton 2012)

(2) Rachel Joyce: The Unlikely Pilgrimage of Harold Fry (Black Swan 2012)

(3) Charles Dickens: Little Dorrit. (1857)

(4) Ben Quash: Abiding (Bloomsbury 2012)

(5) Peter Ackroyd: Albion The Origins of the English Imagination (Vintage 2004)

II
Down South

I am from the North, in Stuart Maconie's phrase the land of "pies and prejudice." (1) Where is that? "Surrounded on two sides by land, on two by sea, existing below Scotland, which is another north altogether, and above the rest of England, above where the south has become the amorphous midlands, which itself, in fits and starts, over rivers, in buildings, in my mind, across fences, becomes the north." (2) I have lived now for a quarter of a century in Cheshire which some people argue is not really part of the north, more a kind of colonial outpost of the Home Counties. Perhaps they are right. However I was born in Manchester, and one of my early memories is of walking to infant school through a "Pea souper" of 1950s smog. Mum had been brought up in Ardwick, a working class area of the city. I recall going as a child to visit her sister and brother-in-law who lived in the same street where mum had spent her childhood. I picture Uncle Phil crouched in front of a tiny black-and-white television set checking his pools coupon, whilst Auntie Ada always seemed to be brewing gallons of tea for the adults. Dad's childhood had been spent in several diffe-rent Lancashire towns as his father was moved to different posts within the Lancashire Constabulary. Dad ended up spen-ding time at three different grammar schools: Blackburn, Bacup and Rawtenstall and Leigh. Grandma and Taid (thence the Welsh blood in me) eventually settled in Droylsden, south of Manchester. Here Grandma lived into her second century, rarely missing an episode of Coronation Street.

So, early life in Manchester – You can't understand the place Manchester United hold in my affections unless you have heard the story of my dad returning from work and telling me that people were weeping openly in the streets as news of the Munich air disaster broke. A passion for sport obviously began very early because the older boys on the street nicknamed me "Cricketing Clarence" as the five-year-old Evans was always desperate to be included in their street cricket.

When I was seven we moved to Nelson, a town in north east Lancashire, and it was here that much of my growing up and formation were done. The immediate reason for the move was that dad got a job as food chemist for the sweet firm Victory V – of lozenges, gums and jelly babies fame. Part of me feels that mum never fully came to terms with leaving Manchester, despite eventually becoming Mayoress of Nelson and later Pendle, its new identity after local government reorganisation. I wonder if that was one factor in the unhappiness which was rarely far from the surface of her life.

Nelson's primary reason for existence had been as a weaving town within the great Lancashire textile industry. Much of that was in terminal decline by the time I arrived on the scene but I recall summer moments watching the activity in the weaving sheds when the huge doors had been left open to allow the fresh air in. When early July brought the traditional wakes weeks (Nelson holidays), the town really did feel deserted. Lines of people queued to catch excursion trains to Blackpool, Morecambe or North Wales. Meanwhile for those who remained in the town there was only a very sketchy local bus service and mum used to complain with a bit of exaggeration that it was difficult even to get hold of a loaf of bread.

A Lancashire childhood in the 1960s was fundamental in forming me. I recall plenty of flat caps though very few clogs. Lines of terraced houses running up and down hillsides. Once you left the main roads many of the side streets retained their original cobbles. There really was a stall on the open market which sold tripe and little else. Primary schooling in an old Victorian building really did see boys and girls separated into separate yards for playtime. We used to chant "who wants to play chain tig, no girls allowed" which was rather redundant really as all the girls were on the far side of an eight foot high stone wall.

Our home was actually on the edge of town with a view across to Pendle Hill, famous for witches and the tradition of climbing it after chapel on Good Friday. On the other side of the cinder track which served as a road there were fields and beyond that disused slate quarries to explore. We had regular run-ins with the local farmer who, with the benefit of hindsight, must have been a great deal more tolerant than we realised. Every winter saw crowds of us sledging (we never called it tobogganing) down a steep field to a frozen stream which awaited the unwary or over adventurous. I was a member of the Trent Road Gang. Our most important time of the year was the period running up to 5th November when we had to guard our "plot" (bonfire) against raids from other gangs who might steal wood or worse still set the bonfire alight prematurely. Honesty requires that I report that we were rather a wimpish lot compared to the gangs from Ringstone Crescent or Rowland Avenue.

We were a strongly Methodist family. Chapel and then afternoon Sunday School whether I liked it or (quite frequently) not. Dad was secretary for our very large Sunday School; on more than one occasion a special train was used for the annual outing to the seaside. Becoming stranded at the top of the big wheel on the fairground when I should have been back at the station to catch the train home led to major parental recriminations. I still feel a lingering sense of injustice about this: it was not my fault that the fairground ride has decided to break down whilst I was swinging gently in midair! At least having a father holding office in the Sunday School meant I was very likely to get a first prize when the books were handed out; anything much less than full attendance meant that you were demoted to a second prize or worse. The chapel had a strong commitment to youth work within a fairly narrow evangelical ethos. As teenagers we not only benefited from the organised activities; we were also allowed to hang out informally on the premises on most evenings of the week.

Looking back, I guess that we were on the cusp between a northern chapel culture which was passing away and the huge changes which the 1960s would bring about (although it was probably rather later that some of the latter impacted on northeast Lancashire). It has been argued strongly that it was this period that saw the biggest collapse in traditional church attendance and Christian commitment. (3) The days when one's entire social and cultural life – whether chapel concert, Wesley Guild, women's meeting or youth fellowship – as well as Sunday worship revolved around the church were numbered. Concert memories include the Cub and Scout gang shows, riding along on the crest of a wave. In one variety show some of us performed a sketch which saw us dressed as "pygmies" singing a song which I believe was entitled "I bent my assegai." Less than fond memories of something that was not only cringingly awful but also undoubtedly racist! It was felt to be very funny and certainly raised no eyebrows in a north-east Lancashire church circa 1965. The town centre church I attended had a congregation of several hundred and in addition to the chapel a huge suite of ancillary buildings including three large halls, a stage, sundry lounges and meeting rooms and even a snooker room. It now uses much smaller redeveloped premises shared with the Roman Catholics and there are many more Moslems than Methodists in its neighbourhood.

So I am a northerner, a Lancashire lad and stubbornly proud of it. Like St Paul in the Letter to the Philippians, I can boast of my background; unlike him I am unwilling to call it all "mere refuse!" (4) Rather: "A human life, I think, should be well rooted in some spot of a native land, where it may get the love of tender kinship for the face of earth, for the labours men go forth to, for the sounds and accents that haunt it, for whatever will give that early home a familiar unmistakable difference amidst the future widening of knowledge that – - -" (5)

To me the North / South divide is so obvious as to be virtually self-evident. The historian Tristram Hunt argues that it had its roots in the first part of the twentieth century and at least in economic terms was exacerbated by Thatcherism. The decline both of the great traditional industries and of Nonconformity was matched by an increasing superiority both in economic and cultural terms of London and the South East. The great civic pride of the northern cities took a tremendous battering and often what remained looked suspiciously like inverted snobbery.

"With London's 20th-century supremacy came a renewed cultural arrogance. "All England is in a suburban relation" to London, declared the novelist Henry James as early as 1905. And the succeeding hundred years saw only an acceleration of that deleterious trend. The corporate and financial stampede southward was quickly followed by the political parties, the media, the professional establishment, the cultural elite, even the representatives of organised labour." (6)

Paul Morley by contrast puts the origins a great deal earlier, to the Norman conquest following 1066. There was, he argues, a southerly shift in political and ecclesiastical power and the beginnings of different systems of cultural and social organisation. From this emerged the notion that some parts of the country were more advanced and important than others, and indeed more sophisticated compared with those up north who were a little backward because of their geographical separation from the spheres of influence. Previously it had made more sense to see England in terms of east and west; now north and south began to assume greater significance in people's minds.

Whatever its historical roots, it meant that a journey down south was a journey into a different country. A mixture of northern pride and northern insecurity accompanied me down the M6 and M1. My university experience took me only as far south as Birmingham but for several terms I was convinced that those who had travelled to the Midlands from the Home Counties were an intellectual cut above me. Posh accents meant their owners were all de facto more intelligent than me (and no doubt some of them were). Those who imagined that civilisation had its boundary at Watford Gap had an effortless superiority when it came to patronising those of us who had been brought up in the midst of the dark satanic mills. Conversely, everyone from down south was simply cosy, affluent, comfortable, perhaps a little effete. Much in need of some experience of the real life that was to be found up north. Just look at how your average metropolitan dweller was thrown into a panic by the arrival of a few winter snow flakes in Surrey or Middlesex.

All this of course bore only a passing relation to reality. But for this prejudiced northerner, it makes sense to use down south as a metaphor for the cosy, the bland and the faintly self-satisfied. Unfair but helpful! But when we come to apply the metaphor, is it altogether unfair to see cosy and bland as a description of much of British church life? This is not to deny even for a moment that the church contains some wonderful caring Christian people. I have met lots of them. Yet from collective church life something feels to be missing. I long for a combination of imagination, passionate commitment and intellectual coherence and find it all too rarely. Cultural analysts focusing on religion detect a variety of developments in the "post-modern" period including a new interest in religious experience and different styles of spirituality, a new awareness of the need to hear a variety of different voices not just the powerful and a new recognition of how complex Christian living can be in a plural society. Thankfully all those things can be found at different places within the church. Sadly all of them appear to be missing from great swathes of it. We are accustomed to the discussion about the gap between the academy and the church pew. It seems to be equally true that there is a large gap between many contemporary theological insights and what I hear regularly from the pulpit. This has nothing to do with any kind of rather dry intellectualism. It is about a longing to hear more preaching which combines an aversion to comfortable cliché, some knowledge of contemporary thinking and a lively enthusiasm in exploring what discipleship of Jesus might involve. Is this too much to ask? "The dreadful thing about so much theology is that, in relation to the reality of the human situation, it is so superficial. Theological categories (really mere theological formulae) are "aimed" without sufficient depth of understanding at life insensitively misunderstood." (7)

It may be this is symptomatic of something much wider which John Hull summarises in trenchant fashion:

"Perhaps we could even say that a fundamental distinction can be made between churches and individual Christians: the theology of power, supremacy, uniqueness and prosperity is one form taken by the Christian faith today, and the theology of brokenness is its principal alternative. The theology of brokenness offers the church a way of replacing the oppressive monolith of an unambiguous perfection with the rich and varied ambiguity of many forms of human brokenness." (8)

If those two alternatives represent the two extremes of the spectrum, I suspect that when you scratch us most of us and the churches we belong to are nearer to the former than the latter. We prefer to be "down south" in our comfort zone! We unconsciously accept the values of consumer and celebrity culture and rarely perceive the message of Jesus and the Kingdom as encouraging us to hear a radically different narrative and to live within it. This is what John Drane has called the McDonaldization of the church – the presentation of its life and message in bland, prepackaged, predictable terms. (9) Our theology and practice alike are in captivity. We like a God who reigns but not one who reigns from a tree on Calvary.

We like a God who intervenes in some circumstances and not others. This is the thrust of many of our prayers both liturgically and in private. But for many years I have wrestled with the notion of an interventionist God who appears to respond arbitrarily to requests for help. I struggle to accept that either intellectually or morally. More and more frequently, I wrestle with believing in a God who is a supreme being outside the life of creation yet somehow directly involved at certain points and in certain moments. I find myself very much in sympathy with this analysis: "This is the God that is still all too current in many contemporary church circles: a personal, external, superperson who intervenes in the lives of particular individuals at times of stress and despair to fix problems. God is the ultimate Fixer of a malfunctioning world machine." (10) Where does that leave me as a Christian? I will explore in a later chapter in what ways I still want to make use of the word God and all that it symbolises. For now I want to note that the onset of physical disability has brought some of these issues into much sharper focus.

The impact on me of those writing theology from the perspective of disability as well as those exploring the nature of disability / impairment has been enormous. Insights that I have been groping incoherently towards for ages have gained a greater clarity. Unexamined assumptions lurking in the shadows have had a new spotlight shone upon them. All this is one of the results of the enforced move from an able-bodied world to a disabled world. Theology from a perspective of disability (alongside writing which engages theological issues in the light of gender, race, sexuality and so on) has a distinctive and important contribution to make. I tried to explore how this might be true particularly in relation to the situation of the traditional British church in my book *Disabled Church?* (11)

Back in the early 1970s Methodist ministerial students were invited to grapple with John Macquarrie's *Principles of Christian Theology.* (12) Many of us found it completely baffling; small wonder when it included sentences such as "Being is more beingful than any being that it lets be." Forty years later I did not have to look up that quotation; it is seared on my consciousness! I did recently take the book down from the shelf and found some of it still very difficult to grasp. Although it is interesting to see how Macquarrie combines extensive use of Martin Heidegger's philosophy with a traditional Anglo-Catholic outlook.

But what if "letting be" is a helpful description of the creative process? Echoing the Genesis creation story repeated pronouncement "Let there be – - -." What if the central quality of the divine is not omnipotence or many of the other traditional attributes of God? What if on the contrary we should look to themes such as self giving, precariousness and vulnerability as the marks of authentic divine love? (13) Of course these are not brand-new themes emerging from nowhere. What does appear to be new is the exploration by some theologians of the idea of a "disabled God." (14) At the crucial weekend for Christian faith, we see Jesus helpless and vulnerable on the cross and then we see a risen Lord – who still bears the marks of his suffering. The body of the risen Lord is impaired! Indeed it is to the marks of impairment that Thomas is directed during his Eastertide encounter with Jesus. One of the implications is that the risen Christ is "a symbol ripe for subversive reclamation and reworking by people with disabilities." (15) Consider the implications of thinking not only that God understands and shares in our disability but also that disability is actually essential to understanding God's nature of love. An end to the long history of speculating whether there are links between disability and sinfulness. An end to thinking that holiness and being without impairment belong together. An end to wondering whether the failure to be given a miracle cure must somehow or other be linked to a lack of faith. Instead, the awareness that disability is not a barrier to reflecting the imago Dei in human life. On the contrary, it may be that people with disabilities can reveal profound aspects of the divine. Not of course because we have any inherent virtue but simply because of the challenge we inherently offer to bracketing godliness with efficiency, autonomy or market value.

Theology and discipleship from the perspective of disability have much to contribute to the understanding and practice of the Christian community. Let two quotations illustrate the possibilities and difficulties inherent in that. The first from a World Council of Churches report:

"We have gifts to share that have emerged precisely from the experience of living with disability – - – We have found ourselves in that liminal space between what is known and what is yet unknown, able only to listen and wait. We have faced fear and death and know our own vulnerability. We have met God in that empty darkness, where we realised we were no longer "in control" and learned to rely on God's presence and care. We have learned to accept graciously and to give graciously, to be appreciative of the present moment. We have learned to negotiate a new terrain, a new way of life that is unfamiliar. We have learned to be adaptable and innovative, to use our imaginations to solve new problems. We can be resilient. We know what it is to live with ambiguity and in the midst of paradox, that simplistic answers and certitudes do not sustain us." (16)

And the difficulties?

In the Church "Power lies with the healthy and the well, and those who are sick are positioned, in structural terms, in a relatively powerless position. This is so in practical terms – - – but also in philosophical terms (whose interpretation of the world and its meaning are taken as normative) – - – To what extent the normatively "well" community is willing to be changed by the experience of those who are ill, or of those who have disabilities. The lived experience of those who have passed from one category to the other is that the Christian community's ability to be so changed is strictly limited. Models of professional ministry, for instance, assume a level of activity and mobility that only the normatively well and able-bodied can attain. Those who had been normatively well but have become ill or developed disabilities have found that the institution finds it impossible to work with their new limitations but also – perhaps more significantly – to accommodate the new insights and gifts to which they feel their new experience gives them access. They find themselves on the margins where once they were the centre." (17)

Little room or justification then for sitting comfortably drinking southern comfort! Insights from the thinking of a theology of disability as well as the lived experience of people with a variety of impairments have much to contribute to Christian communities whose outlook is still very frequently "ableist."

(1) Stuart Maconie: Pies and Prejudice (Ebury Press 2008)

(2) Paul Morley: The North (And Almost Everything in It) (Bloomsbury 2013)

(3) Callum Brown: The Death of Christian Britain Understanding Secularisation 1800-2000 (Routledge 2001)

(4) Philippians 3: 7-8

(5) George Eliot: Daniel Deronda (1876)

(6) Tristram Hunt: Building Jerusalem The Rise and Fall Of the Victorian City (Phoenix paperback edition 2005)

(7) David Jenkins, quoted in David Jasper: The Sacred Desert Religion, Literature, Art And Culture (Blackwell 2004)

(8) John Hull: "The Broken Body In a Broken World A Christian Contribution To a Christian Doctrine Of the Person From a Disabled Point of View," in Journal Of Religion, Disability And Health Volume 7 Number 4 2003

(9) John Drane: The McDonaldization Of the Church (Darton, Longman and Todd 2000)

(10) Sally McFague: The Body of God An Ecological Theology (SCM 1993)

(11) Graham Evans: Disabled Church? (Church In the Marketplace Publications 2010)

(12) John Macquarrie: Principles Of Christian Theology (SCM 1966)

(13) The three key marks of God's love explored by W H Vanstone: Love's Endeavour Love's Expense The Response of Being to the Love of God (Darton, Longman and Todd 1977)

(14) See especially Nancy Eiesland: The Disabled God Towards a Liberatory Theology of Disability (Abingdon Press, 1994)

(15) Lisa Isherwood and Elizabeth Stuart: Introducing Body Theology (Sheffield Academic Press 1998)

(16) Arne Fritson and Samuel Kabue: Interpreting Disability A Church Of All and For All (World Council of Churches Publications 2004)

(17) Alison Webster: Wellbeing (SCM 2002)

III
Out West

The Pesthouse, a novel by Jim Crace, (1) portrays a dystopian vision of America following a plague pandemic resulting in the collapse of civilisation. The main characters journey through a desolate landscape of ruined cities and industries encountering wild robber gangs and devotees of strange religious cults. They are aiming to travel to the coast from where they hope to escape from America altogether. Interestingly it is the Atlantic coast they are moving towards. They are travelling east rather than west which feels counterintuitive. The American dream, the American self understanding and mythology, has always been about going west.

My own journey westwards only took me as far as New York but to be there if only for a week was one of the most remarkable experiences of my life. To stand on the top floor of the World Trade Centre in amazement would prove to be a deeply poignant moment for me is the light of later events on 9/11. But the call to adventure or escape has been: Go West Young man! And countless people have. As the inscription on the Statue of Liberty has it: "Give me your tired, your poor, / Your huddled masses, yearning to breath free, / The wretched refuse of your teeming shore, / Send these, the homeless, tempest tost to me."

Fleeing famine or persecution. Irish, Jewish, Italians, arriving on Ellis Island, being processed and then admitted to New York City and from there gradually spreading out across the country. Always going west – from the early pioneers with their wagon trains to Steinbeck's Okies escaping the dust bowl travelling to California; from the restless youngsters Dean and Sal in Jack Kerouac's *On The Road* to Paul Simon: "So we bought a pack of cigarettes and Mrs Wagner pies / And walked off to look for America." The Chinese immigrant Lee says "We are all descended from the restless, the nervous, the criminals, the arguers and brawlers, but also the brave and independent and generous. If our ancestors had not been that, they would have stayed in their home plots in the other world and starved over the squeezed-out soil." (2)

To travel out west was to discover a new identity for yourself on the journey, to carve out a new space in which to live, to discover who you were and who you might become, to have the freedom in which a rugged individualism and independence could flourish with self-reliance as the watchword. Oh Brave New World that has such people in it! That mythology still holds a powerful resonance in the United States. It helps to explain the deep-seated reluctance to introduce gun control laws, something deeply puzzling to many Europeans. It has fostered a suspicion of federal government. Often it has been in deep tension with other American aspirations – for greater social justice, and civil rights; for collective action whether in industrial relations or in fighting discrimination. These competing visions could be clearly identified in the comparison between the outlook of President Obama and that of The Tea Party.

Of course, going west has not been without its dark side (paramountly in the fate suffered by Native Americans). *On Canaan's Side* proves to be a deeply ironic title for a novel by Sebastian Barry in which the protagonists discover that America is far from being the promised land for which they had dreamed. (3) The elderly narrator tells of how she had to flee from Ireland to America under threat of death because of her relationship with a member of the Black and Tans in the 1920s. But even in the land of milk and honey there is tragedy – the man is murdered by a Republican assassin, and her life is entangled with issues of racial identity and war. Her son and grandson both return – from Vietnam and Iraq respectively – severely traumatised by their experiences.

The journey west can be rooted in the desire to escape painful or threatening circumstances and find a new life. Less dramatically it involves moving outside one's comfort zone in order to discover identity and direction for living – education, career, finding a partner, being a parent – all these mean leaving behind the comforts of home. If I understand him correctly, these are partly what the American Franciscan Richard Rohr describes as the necessary tasks of the first half of life. (4) They are reflected in many of the great mythological stories – Odysseus leaving Ithaca for the Trojan War and his many adventures on the way home – and in the biblical narratives – Abraham setting out for a new country, disciples leaving their nets. Journeying to explore who we are and who we are intended to be.

Rather more mundanely, to put it mildly, what did it mean for a Lancashire lad to leave the comforts of home in my little town in search of an identity? From the age of eleven it meant a train journey five days a week through such exotic stations as Burnley Barracks, Rose Grove and Church and Oswaldtwistle. I had won a scholarship to Queen Elizabeth's Grammar School in Blackburn (in later years I was to wonder how appropriate it was for a local authority to provide funding to access a rather elite institution). Dad was particularly keen for me to go there as he had briefly been a schoolboy there himself. Queen Elizabeth's was a direct grant grammar school with more than a hint of public school ethos about it. A venerable institution, it celebrated its "quatercentenary" during my time there. We sang the school song written in doggerel Latin and at the end of it shouted Vivat! and threw our caps into the air. It was of course an all boys affair. Prefects had a great deal of power to discipline younger boys including their own prefects' detention. Sadly by the time I had the opportunity in that exalted status, the winds of change had begun to blow and the prefects had much less authority so that my chances to prove for myself that power corrupts were more limited. School was divided into six houses named after Elizabethan adventurers some of whom had been no better than they ought to have been – Drake and Raleigh, Howard and Hawkins, Grenville and Frobisher. I was a member of the last named, regular no hopers especially in the area of sporting prowess. There were of course very strong positive elements in this tradition. It provided me with an excellent academic education, almost assisting me to get into Cambridge until I messed up the entrance exams. Many of the staff represented a long tradition of service to a style of education that had nurtured them and in which they strongly believed.

As I write this, the school website carries the obituary of a teacher who had first been there as a pupil and after university returned as a member of staff and later deputy head for some 35 years. To serve them all my days indeed. Nor was everything set in petrified stone. During my final terms I was allowed to teach some English lessons, quite unsupervised, to the first years and introduced my charges to the lyrics of Bob Dylan. I think this rather Bohemian experiment would not be allowed these days!

Nonetheless, there were drawbacks. Where I gained academically, I suffered somewhat socially. It was difficult to take part in after-school activities when home was a fifteen mile train ride away. Nelson and Blackburn had different annual holidays so that I was quite frequently making the usual trek when my friends from Nelson schools were on holiday. In retrospect the all-male environment was a distinct disadvantage: I suffered from painful shyness with girls in my teenage years which co-education would surely have helped to mitigate. I left with a fistful of O-levels and A-levels, a place at a redbrick university and an ability to think which school life especially in the sixth form had enabled to develop but without the necessary confidence to transfer easily into a wider social world.

Meanwhile, there had been significant developments in my involvement with the Methodist Church. My first experiences in leading worship and preaching were as a member of a "youth mission band" of teenagers which led worship at several of the local Methodist churches. I quite often was given the task of reading a mini sermon, partly I suspect because I had a louder than average speaking voice! Kindly Methodists were very supportive and encouraging of our efforts. Here was something that I was good at and everyone told me I was good at it! I basked in the warm glow of praise from those who wanted to affirm what the "Young people" were achieving. I have no doubt that a large percentage of my responding to a "call to preach" was ego driven. God moves in mysterious ways! So it was that I began training as a Local Preacher, becoming fully accredited in 1972 at the age of 20. Much of my early preaching was heavily influenced by the Christian social and political commentary of people like Colin Morris – I remember that his book *Unyoung, Uncoloured, Unpoor* had a particular impact on me and was raided wholesale for some of my sermons. Goodness knows what some in the congregations made of it all; they were probably too polite to say!

The next move metaphorically out west was the beginning of university life in Birmingham, reading for a degree in English and Theology. Like many an undergraduate before and since, the first few terms were far from comfortable with my mixture of shyness and homesickness with which to contend. Communication with the north was of course limited to the occasional phone call from a public box or the occasional letter via Royal Mail – no e-mails, texts, Skype or Facebook! My student life almost came to an abrupt end at the end of the first year but I just about scraped through the exams and was permitted to remain. Having fortunately had this narrow escape, I managed to emerge two years later with an upper

29

second BA degree. Meanwhile, without any fanfare of celestial trumpets, I had begun to think about ordained ministry as the path I should be following. I duly offered as a candidate for the Methodist ministry, was accepted and went straight from university into ministerial training – just around the corner at Queen's College Birmingham.

The Chair of the national committee which was the final hurdle before acceptance for ministerial training gently chided me during my interview because there was rather a lot of politics in my answers whereas the theological content was a little thin. Following on from that recollection, a brief diversion into my political background. An interest in politics was a natural part of family life. We were unquestionably Labour. The first General Election I recall was Harold Wilson's narrow victory in 1964; an excitement which was certainly surpassed by Tony Blair's landslide in 1997. I guess that dad was on the Gaitskellite wing of the party; mum would sometimes irritate him by suggesting he was really a closet liberal. Her own political opinions were much more intuitive, the product of a working-class upbringing in Manchester between the wars. She found it incomprehensible when working people voted Tory. She cheered when Neil Kinnock savaged the Militant Tendency and was prone to say "Get that woman off" whenever Mrs Thatcher appeared on television. Her instinctive commitment to the party even survived the machinations and compromises of New Labour. Dad was much more directly involved, serving for many years as a local councillor and being elected Mayor on two separate occasions. I recall collecting numbers in polling stations, working in committee rooms and "knocking up" to encourage our natural supporters not to forget to vote. This in a town which had in the past been nicknamed by some people "Little Moscow." I think it is true that when we moved there in 1959 the town council was 100% Labour without any opposition parties at all. Not very good for democracy I guess!

Emerging from that background, my own political convictions have become more nuanced but haven't really altered much in their basic orientation. If anything I have become rather more left-wing in recent years in a somewhat unfocused and undisciplined way. The loss of community strikes me as deeply worrying amidst all the stress on individual getting ahead. I hate it when affluent government ministers tell us that we "are all in this together" as a justification for austerity measures which impact disproportionately on the less well off. Volunteering at a local food bank gives me weekly encounters with people at the sharp end of the attack on the poor and disabled. I sense vaguely that capitalism is not producing societies in which we can develop that abundant living which Christian tradition claims is God's intention for us all.

Anyway, back to the student minister. Life at Queen's in the early 1970s was certainly interesting. It had just been launched as an ecumenical college. There were Methodists who had moved there from Handsworth College when it closed to become a partner in the new setup. There were Anglo-Catholics who found themselves there after the closure of their college in Lichfield. There were women in training for the Wesley Deaconess Order. There were theological left-wingers who had been influenced by writing and thinking about the "the death of God." It was certainly lively and challenging, although life in that setting frequently had something of a hothouse feel to it and, despite the beginnings of a new stress on pastoral theology and placements in hospital or community, leafy Edgbaston still had something of the ivory tower about it. The demographics were of course changing with many more students already married whilst in earlier years Methodist ministerial training had been virtually limited to single men. Debates were frequently lively and there were lots of opportunities for cultural and sporting pursuits. I had my only major amateur dramatics role in a play written by one of my fellow students (playing a rather bigoted northern Methodist!). I discovered the joys of squash, tennis and playing for a football team which made up in enthusiasm what it lacked in ability. The team from the lay training centre Cliff College was certainly the most pious we played, gathering for a brief prayer before kick-off. Their tackling was also the keenest we came across!

The period of training was not without its sloughs of despond. A crisis in personal relationships led to me taking "a year out" which I spent working as a labourer in a large timber yard. This brought me into contact with men whose lifestyle and opinions were quite different than any I had previously encountered. And, at the risk of sounding very corny or like a sentimental socialist of the worst kind, I really enjoyed manual labour. However, at the end of the year I returned to the ecclesiastical fray and was ordained in 1979. In the first church in which I was "stationed" I met Becky and we were married in 1981.

I'm not sure how far I moved out of my comfort zone in fulfilling these first half of life tasks. But it looked as though a fairly strong identity had either been given or worked out: a northern nonconformist, grammar school and university educated, left-wing in opinions, ordained in my vocation as a Methodist minister, in a married relationship which I assumed would be for a lifetime and with the enjoyable prospect of becoming a parent on the horizon. The latter hope was to be realised as the father of two daughters and a son. The following years inevitably were not without difficulties, some of which

I allude to in later pages. However for the moment I want to fast forward to the early years of the new millennium and describe briefly how several aspects of that identity took a severe battering.

In 2000, after a battery of tests including the delights of MRI scans and a lumbar puncture, I was diagnosed with Primary Progressive Multiple Sclerosis. The situation developed quite rapidly and I soon needed to make use of a wheelchair. By 2004 I felt that there was little option but to apply for early retirement on disability grounds which was duly granted. That year was probably my annus horribilis as it also included several lengthy stays in hospital. Just to complete the picture of those years my marriage came to an end and my wife and I separated in 2006. Whilst it would be mistaken to assume that the onset of disability led to the breakup (relationships are surely more complex than that), I think that things would not have happened in quite the same way without it.

There is quite frequent conversation in the MS community about how it is presented in the media. Some feel it is relentlessly upbeat whilst others feel that the focus is far too negative. It seems to me that an honest understanding demands a straightforward account of the difficulties to begin with. "Many disabled adults do not have the right to decide what time to get up or go to bed, or indeed who to go to bed with, when or what to eat, how often to bath or even be in control of the times when they empty their bladders or open their bowels." (5) That sounds like me. There is both frustration and humiliation on a daily basis. My body is nonconformist and I have an ambivalent relationship with it – probably more aware of it than I have ever been but at the same time angry with it. At a very basic physical level the move into being a person with disabilities has involved an attack on my identity.

Beyond that, key elements in making up who I am have taken a beating. I thought I would be in full-time Methodist ministry until I was 65 but that active vocation has gone. To move from being a Superintendent minister into early retirement is to move from the centre to the margins. I am aware that many retired ministers say similar things; it just happened rather earlier and more abruptly for me. I felt a little like Superman in the comic books popping into a telephone box and emerging as Clark Kent! I imagined that I was in a lifelong marital relationship with all its ups and downs but that has come to an end. Dreams of what might be done in later retirement have been dashed: climbing all the Lake District fells (feasible); buying a camper van and criss-crossing the United States in it (feasible if I had won the lottery). On holiday a few years back I was at the end of one of the long peninsulas which make up the coastline of south-west Ireland. It was a late June evening and I looked out over the Atlantic at the sun going down in the general direction of the Americas. To get a better photograph I tried to get onto a small grassy hillock next to the car. It took all my energy and bloody mindedness to do it. A few years before I would have expended less energy in walking to the summit of one of the larger mountain peaks in Cumbria or Scotland. Now even the summit of the hillock would be out of reach.

But more needs to be said than just an account of these rather crippling (!) blows. Not in terms of discovering silver linings amongst the clouds although there have been some of those. Nor in terms of living daily in the hope of a cure. I would of course take one if it was offered – I am not a masochist, still less a saint. But I cannot relate to the world of miracle / faith healings with integrity. I find much of both its theology and its ethics problematic, not to mention pastorally insensitive. Moreover, constantly looking for that kind of escape route can mean constantly finding yourself in a cul-de-sac. Such dead ends are not helpful in the tasks of living life as a person with disabilities. For me it makes more sense to ask myself what I can hope for and how I might build a framework of meaning in my new circumstances. In this area I have found the writing of the theologian and educationalist John Hull, who himself went blind in his adult years, particularly stimulating. (6)

For Hull, the generally accepted position is that there is one "normal" world which is inhabited by the able-bodied and from which to one degree or another those with disabilities are excluded. Instead he posits a plurality of different worlds each with its own distinctive characteristics. This is perhaps particularly evident in his own situation of blindness but it applies to a wide range of conditions involving sensory, mobility or learning impairments.

"If someone is born into a disabled condition, the world generated by that state is formed from the earliest days. One is, so to speak, born a citizen of that world. On the other hand, if one becomes disabled at a later stage, whether during childhood or in adult life, one experiences the shock of losing one's world." (7)

So, someone like me becoming disabled is, in some kind of population relocation, forced to move from one world to another. There are of course continuities between the two. I can of course look back regretfully to the able-bodied world. Ralf, a man gradually losing his sight, is consciously doing that: "Before blindness erased his world he was determined to draw up an inventory of things he wished to study, to furnish his blind world with. He was like a traveller packing for a long journey. He had to decide which memories and knowledge of things he wished to take into this new world he was headed for." (8)

I can also end up so consumed with regrets and bitterness that I am constantly looking back over my shoulder. However, the invitation is to be born again into this new world and to discover creative ways of living in it. And it is certainly true that all sorts of people, experiences and events look different from a permanent seat in a wheelchair.

"The recently disabled person either renounces the old world and accepts the new, now disabled body, or on the other hand refuses to let the old world go, insists on continuing to try to live within it, and perhaps longs and prays for the miracle which will restore not just the former body but the former world. The painful choice is made more poignant by the fact that since the everyday world of the average person is not conscious of its distinctive character as a world but imagines itself to be the only reality, the newly disabled person cannot imagine any other world than the one he or she has now left. The normal world regards the disabled person as banished, excluded, deprived as it were of citizenship rights, and as therefore to be pitied and helped." (9)

Imagining this multiplicity of worlds has lots of consequences. It helps combat the view of disability which sees it only in terms of deficiency and exclusion. Our understanding of what it means to be human is extended. Respect for difference is encouraged. Hull sees this as having a potentially subversive effect in that it can help to highlight other claims to be an absolute – whether in religion, economic systems or attitudes to gender or race issues. However it must be said that both Bible and Christian tradition are frequently unhelpful. Take the traditional Christian metanarrative. There were no disabilities in the Garden of Eden and there will be none in the renewed creation: "Then will the lame leap like the deer and the mute tongue shout for joy." (10) So disability belongs to the fallen world in need of redemption. This approach may not be so crass as to imagine that individual disability is the result of individual sinfulness (although there are more than a few examples of that in the pages of the Bible). Yet disability seems to be linked with disease, natural disaster and all those factors which seem to mitigate against the Genesis creation claim that God looked on everything he had made and it was very good. It remains of course to ask the question which I will come back to in subsequent pages about whether there are other elements in the Christian tradition which are more helpful in constructing a "disabled theology."

Enough has been said already to indicate that relationships between people with disabilities and those who are temporarily able-bodied are about attitudes as well as architecture. The provision of a loop system, large print books and ramps is excellent but only a small part of the story. John Hull tells of visiting a church for the disabled in South Korea. When asked why they needed a separate church, the members replied that they had no choice since their attendance at "normal" church made the able-bodied feel uncomfortable. That route seems an exceptional one. Yet those of us with disabilities can create embarrassment and uncertainty in others who don't know quite how to relate to us. I am never approached in the street or the supermarket and asked if I would like to consider changing my energy supplier or whether I have been mistakenly sold payment protection insurance (this could be construed as one of life's blessings!). If I make an enquiry in a shop or at the reception desk in the dentist's, the reply will often be directed to my carer even though I have done the initial speaking. Within a specifically Christian context, we raise awkward questions about faith or lack of it, cure or lack of it, well-being or lack of it. Alternatively we are valorised unrealistically as wonderful examples of how to cope with adversity.

What seems to be missing too often is the asking of questions such as: How can the wider Christian community learn from the perspectives of people with disabilities? How might the understanding of major Christian themes be changed and enriched by a theology of disability? The Methodist Conference in 2013 received a report entitled *Supporting Ministers with Ill-health* which contained a section on the support of those with disabilities or impairments. There was much careful and helpful advice about what could and should be done for people in those situations. What I missed was any attempt to establish a context of asking what particular and unique contributions might be made to the understanding of ministry and discipleship by those with disabilities. Perhaps this was not part of the remit. Perhaps it should have been – such a recognition would contribute significantly to the sense of well-being of those who might feel their distinctive contributions are overlooked or ignored.

So here I am in this new world which I had no inkling I would ever have to join and definitely didn't want to. Perhaps like Jesus I have been driven into the wilderness by the Spirit. But I am not finding it easy. On the Sunday before I wrote this, the final hymn in the morning service invited God to "give us courage to choose again the pilgrim way." My ability to drive my powered wheelchair was particularly poor that morning and a journey home which should have taken about ten minutes took over half an hour of frustrated stopping and starting. I wondered how many others in the congregation were having such an immediate and bodily encounter with difficulties on the pilgrim way.

I speculate that people who become blind or profoundly deaf have a much more dramatic move into a new world than mine. Nevertheless, living with progressive MS has impacted on identity, vocation, sexuality, expectations and dreams. Not to mention the stiff neck which I get from constantly talking to people who are standing whilst I am sitting! I am too old to be going out west again; perhaps there will be other ways of discovering what I am now meant to be.

(1) Jim Crace: The Pesthouse (Picador 2007)

(2) John Steinbeck: East of Eden (1952)

(3) Sebastian Barry: On Canaan's Side (Faber and Faber 2011)

(4) Richard Rohr: Falling Upward (Jossey-Bass 2011)

(5) Michael Oliver: Understanding Disability From Theory to Practice (Macmillan 1996)

(6) John Hull, see especially "Spirituality of Disability The Christian Heritage As Both Problem And Potential" Studies In Christian Ethics, volume 16 no 2 2003

(7) Hull: "Spirituality of Disability"

(8) Lloyd Jones: Hand Me Down World (John Murray 2011)

(9) Hull: "Spirituality of Disability"

(10) Isaiah 35: 6

IV
Downtown

In the autumn of 1981, much to my surprise, I found myself learning how to be a coach driver. The location was the St Anns area of inner-city Nottingham and I had just been "stationed" there for my first appointment after ordination. The church owned a thirty seater coach and operated a community transport scheme as a vital part of its work. Equally it was an important part of the minister's role to drive it, not to mention raise funds to keep it on the road. Never having driven anything larger than a Ford Escort before, much blood, sweat and tears were involved through a particularly hot September but eventually I began to master the skill. And to enjoy pretending to be a professional coach driver. We did have one or two other volunteer drivers and later were to employ someone with funds from a government community programme scheme. But over the next few years a lot of time was spent picking up the elderly to take them to "Grub Club", taking disadvantaged youngsters on holiday to North Devon or transporting wives and families of prisoners to visit Lincoln prison. It was enormously satisfying too to raise funds to purchase a new and better vehicle. It became the standard joke to say that if I had to choose between selling the church and selling the bus, the church would have to go!

I had asked for an inner-city appointment and got what I wanted. St Anns had been a traditional inner-city working-class area, a neighbourhood which sociologists had written about. (1) During the 1960s much of it had been demolished with a large number of low rise flats and maisonettes replacing the old terraces. The perceived wisdom amongst the locals who remembered the old St Anns was that, whilst the housing was now better, everything else was worse, particularly the much diminished sense of community and the dearth of local shops and facilities. The Methodist Church did in fact have three small shops incorporated into its premises, providing a vital source of rental income. There had been a Methodist

Church in the area since the early 1880s although the building which was the base for my work had only taken its present form when it was rebuilt in the post-war years, a German incendiary bomb having caused a large amount of wartime damage.

Whilst my theological training had been stimulating, little of it had helped prepare me for this kind of appointment. Lack of bus driving skills was merely the most obvious gap on my CV! Almost everything revolved around the full-time ordained person. The congregation was a mixture of people who for one reason or another had a link with that particular church but now lived in the suburbs, alongside a number of local people. Attempting to foster local leadership was sometimes in tension with the more middle-class Methodists who had traditionally run the church – and whose generous giving was essential to keep it afloat. How do you persuade someone that they have the ability to manage the church books when they see that the previous treasurer was a partner in a large firm of auditors whose secretary produced immaculate accounts at each end of the financial year? One self-made businessman and lifelong Methodist refused to receive Holy Communion from the hands of a local working-class man who had been appointed as a Church Steward on the grounds that the latter was not "good enough" to undertake that role in worship. His interesting theological position was not typical but there was frequently a rather large gap in expectation and understanding between the Sunday congregation and many of those who attended the midweek activities.

Much of this meant me travelling up a steep learning curve. Nevertheless, I threw myself heart and soul into the work. I now see that I did that to such an extent that I neglected my wife and young family. If I had my time over again I would certainly spend a bit less of it working! Not only was I working in a difficult area, as a family we were living in the same area, less than half a mile from the church. Indeed, one of the things that was noted in a lively lunch forum for professionals working in St Anns was that unlike the social workers, health visitors, teachers and so on, the clergy were virtually the only ones living there after office hours.

Kings Hall Methodist Church, a missionary outpost of the city centre mission the Albert Hall, was heavily involved in community work. It had a lengthy tradition of open youth work which had been developed in a remarkable way by my predecessor who had a great gift for working with unchurched and often problematic youngsters. Attempting to respond locally to the large numbers of unemployed school leavers which Thatcherite policies had helped to produce, we launched a daytime drop-in centre called 16-UP in conjunction with the local probation service. A job club met on the church premises. Later, with the assistance of a national Methodist fund called Mission Alongside The Poor, we were able to employ someone supervising offenders doing community service work. All this I look back on with some satisfaction. It was interesting and sometimes pioneering ministry but it always existed on a knife edge. As indeed did the whole life of that church. During my time there, we celebrated the church centenary and, with a hubris unrecognised at the time, we called it "The First Hundred Years." Alas, the first hundred years was the last hundred years and the church actually closed only a few years after I had moved on to a new appointment.

Working in St Anns, it was impossible to miss seeing the impact of political decisions on individual people and the patterns of social deprivation being repeated from one generation to another. It was equally impossible to avoid concluding that there were some remarkable people living there. Their names and faces appear out of my memory as I am dictating this and some of them will be mentioned in a later reflection.

Looking back the 1980s was also a time when I saw wider political issues in sharp relief. The lines of argument were more sharply drawn then. You knew where you stood in relation to a variety of emotive issues. I felt deeply that sending a task force into war in the Falkland Islands was wrong, but really could not see what a viable alternative might be. The sinking of the Belgrano produced a real sense not only of sadness but of shame. I was involved with setting up a local welfare rights advice group and it seemed as though at every committee meeting one of the activists would tell me that I should be preaching about HIV/AIDs in every sermon on every Sunday as the spread of that catastrophe became evident. There was much protest about the stationing of American Cruise missiles in Britain. The Campaign for Nuclear Disarmament enjoyed a great increase in membership and encouraged people to set up neighbourhood groups. The St Anns group met in the Methodist Church. Sometimes there were only three of us. One regular attender went on to become a Labour Member of Parliament. The other was an International Marxist who, scorning the distribution of leaflets or signing of petitions, wanted us to occupy a US air force base. It was never entirely clear how the three of us were going to manage that!

I think that, above all, it was the miners' strike which had a big impact on me. Living in Nottingham I was of course in the midst of the area where the refusal of miners to strike was one of the factors in the failure of the action. Indeed one of my church members was a working miner with a less than flattering opinion of Arthur Scargill. However, you did not need to travel far north of Nottingham to discover police by the vanload stationed to prevent flying pickets from Yorkshire travelling south. If things had worked out differently for me, I could well have been sent as a minister twelve months previously to pit villages on the outskirts of Barnsley and would undoubtedly have seen things from a very different perspective. As it was, it seemed to me that, however many arguments there were about strategy and tactics and however many worries about violence, the destruction of mining communities was both planned and vindictive. A deep sense of community and solidarity was bludgeoned to death. And anyone with the sketchiest knowledge of the history of coal mining in Britain surely winced at the description of miners as part of "the enemy within."

In the midst of the strike in September 1984, I made what should have been an innocuous but turned out to be a fateful journey. I returned to my home church to conduct their harvest festival services. It was meant to be a case of local boy who has made good returns if not in triumph then in a modest amount of glory. All went reasonably well with the worship leading until, in the midst of the evening service, I began to feel seriously unwell – trembling legs, clammy hands and waves of dizziness. I struggled on, managed to complete the service and began to feel rather better. A visit to my GP on the following day produced the suggestion that I was probably suffering from some kind of virus. However, the symptoms recurred in the weeks following, particularly in public speaking situations, although I also began to experience them in other contexts. Eventually I was referred to a consultant who concluded that I was suffering from an anxiety disorder. Perhaps fortunately I had no inkling that this was going to dominate the middle years of my life.

If you imagine a person's anxiety level as the amount of liquid in a bottle, then everyone has some content to the bottle. But if the level is already quite high, then any kind of stressful situation might cause the contents to overflow – this is a panic attack. The symptoms are difficult to describe to anyone who has not experienced them: to me it felt as though dizziness or vertigo led to waves of blackness washing over me. It felt as though I was losing touch with the solidity of the real world around me. I would switch on to some kind of automatic pilot and manage to struggle on until eventually normality was restored. Sometimes after a series of these attacks I would slump into a period of depression which would necessitate having time away from work.

For the next twenty years I never led a Sunday service, conducted a wedding or funeral, or undertook any kind of speaking engagement without the assistance of medication. During that time I was referred for various forms of help. I learned how to score my anxiety levels using the techniques of cognitive behavioural therapy. I was referred for several forms of rather more esoteric counselling whose practitioners all had their own particular analysis. The causes of anxiety were variously identified as repressed anger or the need to relive my earliest days not excluding a recapitulation of my birth experience. I learned a lot about myself but none of it really made me feel any better. The only thing that would deal effectively most of the time with the symptoms was taking tranquillisers in advance of a potentially panic inducing event. Usually that prop would result in a dampening down or suppressing of the panic. I had a complex relationship with the medication: I never took it frequently enough to develop a physical dependency but no doubt there was a psychological dependency on "my little blue pills." I would bite my tongue and keep my counsel when well-meaning but ignorant Christians waxed lyrical about the evils of tranquillisers and how doctors were doling them out like sweets to patients. Without them I would not have been able to sustain my ministry.

I am sure that a great many people from my congregations would have been very surprised to know what was happening to me. Apparently I always gave the impression of being both competent and confident in my worship leading and preaching roles. Those few people with whom I shared something of the situation were frequently at a loss to understand what I was attempting to describe. A senior minister with lots of pastoral experience just said to me in a slightly dismissive way "Of course we all get a little nervous when conducting services Graham." There is of course a world of difference between a healthy nervousness which enhances performance and the levels of anxiety / panic that I was experiencing. The rush of adrenaline produces the fight or flight response in the body but it is impossible to do either when you are marooned as it were in a pulpit, at a lectern or behind a Communion table.

It is only with the benefit of hindsight that I realise how difficult all this must have been for those closest to me in my family. It was often difficult to assume that I would get through any particular day without my bottle of anxiety overflowing. I think back to occasions when one of my young daughters saw me in a state of depression or agitation and must have been puzzled and upset by what was happening to Dad. All too frequently anxiety drives a person into themselves too much, checking their physical symptoms to determine how things are going. The more frequently that panics occur in particular situations, the more likely they are to recur in those situations as the pattern becomes more deeply embedded in one's consciousness. I think that, if I had received expert help right away in September 1984, it might have been possible to nip things in the bud and the next twenty years or so might have felt very different.

One of the issues which perplexed me the most was how the attacks were directed at one of my strengths. I knew that I was a better than average preacher and leader of worship and that I was improving all the time. Indeed, not being blessed with an abundance of false modesty, I was pretty good at it. Yet no strategy seemed to enable me to get back to a situation where I was relaxed and at ease in the public performance of my ministry. In simple terms, why was I feeling so lousy in situations which in theory allowed me to use and develop gifts and talents I had been given? To some extent I am still searching for answers to that question some thirty years later.

The downtown experience was certainly a challenging one. Not only in terms of mental and emotional health and well-being, but also in the questions it raised about the understanding of church and ministry and in opening me up to a wide vista of different people and situations. One of the main factors in deciding to move on was concern about the quality of my children's education. For example, to conduct an assembly at one of the two local comprehensive schools was to enter a severely demoralised environment with a staff struggling heroically against great odds or lapsing into cynicism. Inner city life and ministry were exciting and absorbing but I have to confess that moving to something different did have something in common with stopping banging your head against a brick wall. No doubt John Vincent, whose pioneering work with the Urban Theology Unit influenced many of us, would have said that I was moving from a more real to a less real context for Christian ministry. Actually, at least for a short time, my move to suburban Chester felt like I had embarked on a lengthy holiday! Where had the signs of multiple disadvantage stretching back generations in some families gone? Where were those living in dire situations of relative poverty, limping from one financial crisis to the next? What had happened to all the brown and black faces? On my street in Nottingham there were people whose origins were in Poland, the Ukraine, the Caribbean and the Indian subcontinent. In course of time I discovered that all those people and situations were represented in Chester, but nowhere near as obviously as they had been in St Anns. Over the next few years I heard from afar how the neighbourhood where I had lived had sunk further into problems of drug related violent crime and prostitution. And the Methodist presence which had taken up so much of my energy and commitment to help sustain came to an end.

The difficulties with anxiety and depression made the journey from inner-city to suburbs with me. The little blue tablets remained an essential part of the pattern of life. But very slowly over the years the number of situations in which I felt I needed medicinal assistance and the amount of drugs I was taking began to reduce. More often a pill was swallowed "just in case." Eventually, and I cannot put a precise date on this, the symptoms just seemed to fade away and I have not requested a prescription for tranquillisers for over a decade now.

What had happened to the anxiety and panic attacks? Perhaps I had simply outgrown them with age. No doubt having to retire early from the demands of full-time circuit ministry helped. And in a paradoxical way as the MS developed, so issues of anxiety seemed to reduce. I have pondered that mysterious relationship quite frequently but am no nearer to any kind of satisfactory explanation. Unless of course it is sufficient to say I now really did have something concrete to worry about instead of free-floating, unhealthy panic!

Beyond those specific things, I think that some of the insights I had gained through counselling and had long accepted at a cerebral level had finally penetrated deeply enough into my self- perception to be taken to heart. This was notably true of a false sense of perfectionism within me. From early school days it had been the case that I was expected to come top of the form; coming second or third was deemed to be slightly disappointing. I don't want to give any impression that my parents were unreasonably demanding. They simply wanted me to do well but there was a negative consequence to that as an unhealthy perfectionism gradually seeped into my psyche. So it was that no act of worship I was leading or sermon I was preaching could be a reasonable offering based on the time and effort I had put in in the previous week. Each time I wanted it to be the best I had ever done. Naturally this was setting myself up for failure. Anxiety guaranteed!

As part of the same package of characteristics, I felt that only by performing at this very high level all the time would I be found acceptable in my ministry and in myself. A universal desire to be liked and at a deeper level to be loved became rather skewed into a neurotic compulsion. Only by being at my best and working at my best could I be likeable. There is nothing superficial about all this. On the contrary it relates to some of our deepest primal instincts. I recall once in the midst of a bout of depression someone close to me saying "I don't know what you want me to do for you." My rather anguished response was: "I want you to love me." As I relive that moment years later, I can see that I was in touch with something fundamental and basic to who I am.

It would be a mistake surely for me to assume that those things belong only to my past. The difference seems to be that now I can observe them, look at them, and in recognising their potential impact can reduce their influence. In all this there is wisdom in the words of the Jesuit Anthony de Mello: "Before I was twenty, I never worried about what other people thought of me. But after I was twenty I worried endlessly – about all the impressions I made and how people were evaluating me. Only sometime after turning fifty did I realise that they hardly ever thought about me at all." (2)

Through all this, did I discover that like St Paul with his thorn in the flesh, grace was sufficient? (3) Perhaps I did. There were no moments of peace, tranquillity or harmony in response to prayers. Indeed, I have a long-standing inability to empathise with the words of the hymn "What a friend we have in Jesus." More than that, I confess to a slight feeling of disappointment when I discovered that it had made the cut in the latest Methodist hymn book. But there was a doggedness, a bloody mindedness, a refusal to give up what I considered to be a vocation. Maybe these were the gifts that were given to me. I sometimes felt like one of those toy clowns mounted on a round base which keep popping back up right no matter how often you knock them over. I kept coming back for more and I believe this enabled me to have an effective ministry.

Yet it remains true that, beyond the wariness about mental health issues that still exists in the wider community, the role of priest or minister can bring a sharper focus to the situation. So, nearly thirty years down the line, I am still not entirely sanguine in writing about these problems. Clergy traditionally are not meant to share their weaknesses and vulnerability with the wider church community. Surely the professionally religious have strong enough faith to deal with these things even if surprisingly they suffer from them at all? Jesus said quite clearly "Do not be anxious." (4) Doesn't an anxiety disorder then betoken a lack of faith? These stereotypes certainly infected me. I did not feel able to share aspects of my situation openly with more than a tiny handful of fellow Christians.

In latter years I have come to discover that congregations can actually find it very liberating when the minister / preacher admits to doubts or difficulties. It can be very isolating to feel that you are the only one in a congregation wrestling with doubts and fears. So that it can be a pleasant surprise when the woman or man leading worship is found sometimes to have more questions than answers too. I had a very strong positive response to a sermon which I began with the words "I do wish Jesus hadn't said that." We need much more exploration of Paul's paradoxical reflections on weakness and strength. There is fundamental gospel truth here to which we pay lip service but which needs to occupy a much more central place in our Christian understanding.

An end to perfectionism and the beginning of the recognition that vulnerability and weakness can be the seed beds in which Christian discipleship grows have been crucial developments for me. I find Gospel truth reflected in some lyrics by Leonard Cohen: "Forget your perfect offering / There is a crack in everything / That's how the light gets in." (5) It has taken me a long time to get there and even now I feel I have only just begun to scratch the surface of its truth. Making more of that truth my own will be part of discovering the liberty which is promised to the children of God. (6) It is one key aspect of what it means to be "rooted and grounded in love." (7) Perhaps it is when we begin to come to terms with a neurotic need to be loved that we begin to discover the freedom in which we find we can both love as ourselves and be loved for ourselves.

(1) Ken Coates and Richard Silburn: Poverty The Forgotten Englishmen (1967)

(2) Quoted in Belden Lane: The Solace of Fierce Landscapes (Oxford University Press, 1998)

(3) II Corinthians 12: 7-9

(4) Matthew 6: 25-34

(5) Leonard Cohen: "Anthem"

(6) Romans 8: 21

(7) Ephesians 3: 17

V
Back East

On my coast to coast adventure, I travelled from west to east in line with Wainwright's rather prosaic reasoning that I would then have the prevailing wind at my back. In my case it would not have mattered since I was given a surprising fortnight of quiet, dry weather for my crossing. It was though a journey in some respects from the known to the unknown as I was very familiar with the Lake District fells but knew virtually nothing about the North Yorks Moors.

As a metaphor, travelling eastwards has a certain exotic ring to it (although the reality of Scarborough or Filey stands in rather marked contrast!). Looking east means looking towards the mystic Orient, the land of spices, like Turkish delight full of Eastern promise. There is a long history in the West of fascination with the geography, the life and the religions of the East. In the latter part of the nineteenth century many Westerners were fascinated by Tibet: "To many in the West the country seemed like an icy Eden: an elevated sanctum in the heart of Asia. There the Tibetans led undisturbed lives, in harmony with the rhythms of the dramatic landscape around them, and morally purified by the beauty and thin air." (1) Naturally such romantic notions did not get in the way of the exploitation of India and China and other ancient civilisations. Commerce and Christianity travelled together and then later came empire building, the colonising and subjugation of "the natives" whose good fortune it was to become part of the British Empire.

Nevertheless, when the Beatles went to spend time in India with the Maharishi, it was only their celebrity fame which made the journey appear novel. Perhaps their influence led to an increase in those travelling east to explore the beliefs and practices of Buddhism and Hinduism. But long before Lennon and Harrison, there have been those in the West who have wanted to immerse themselves in one or other aspect of Eastern culture. The novelist Hermann Hesse did just that whilst working on his story *Siddhartha*. Published in 1922, it recounts the journey of self-discovery made by the son of a Brahmin in ancient India. We see Siddhartha variously as a beggar leading an ascetic life, meeting the Buddha, living with a beautiful woman and becoming a successful businessman. Eventually he discovers peace and enlightenment in contemplation by a sacred river. Elements of both Hindu and Buddhist teaching form the philosophical heart of the book and help to interpret Siddhartha's many experiences on his way to inner harmony and wholeness. Interestingly, after being translated into English some thirty years after its original publication, it became something of a cult book during the 1960s amongst young Westerners who were looking back east as one part of the hippie subculture.

Whereas travelling west has a flavour of a vigorous march forwards, the notion of travelling east has a more reflective feel to it. You take the slow train, or perhaps reduce your pace to the speed of the Japanese theologian Koyuke Koyama's "Three mile an hour God" (2) Rather than making your mark on the world, the focus is on exploring your inner nature, a journey in search of your True Self. Not that the two are necessarily incompatible. I am reminded of Charles Darwin, walking the "sand path" which he laid out in the grounds of his home at Down House, thinking thoughts and agonising over their personal implications for him in ways which would change the world.

In mythology, sacred story and literature of course the difficulties and temptations met on the journey are almost always symbolic of the struggles in the inner life of the protagonist.

This appears to be true across many cultures and civilisations. One of the earliest pieces of literature we still possess, which emerged from Mesopotamia many centuries BC, is the *Epic of Gilgamesh*. In epic poetry form, it follows Gilgamesh on his quest in search of immortality. His journey is regularly interspersed with contact with the gods. Similar themes emerge supremely in Homer's *Odyssey* which has arguably had more influence on Western literature than any other single story. As so often in sacred story, the goal of the journey is to return to where the hero started. Thus Odysseus leaves Ithaca to fight in the Trojan Wars and to return home to his wife and son takes a journey of twenty years and involves a host of challenges and difficulties. Parts of the *Odyssey* were used in works as diverse as *The Book of Thousand and One Nights* and Dante's *Inferno*. It provides a structure for James Joyce's great modernist novel *Ulysses* (1922). It influences modern novels / films such as *Cold Mountain* (Charles Frazier 1997) which places the themes in the setting of a man returning home at the end of the American Civil War and the Coen brothers' *O Brother, Where Art Thou?* (2000), a film based loosely around motifs from the *Odyssey*. The breadth of its influence is perhaps best recognised when we learn that it formed the basis of an episode of *The Simpsons* – with Homer Simpson playing the part of Odysseus!

A couple more examples from a vast range of possible sources must suffice. The sixteenth century Chinese classic *Monkey* recounts the travel of Prince Tripitaka and his companions as they seek for enlightenment and the scriptures. Before the writing of the story, the Prince had been a historical character who had made the journey to India and around whom many legends had gathered. Collectively the characters allegorically represent the strengths and weaknesses of humanity. Their journey involves overcoming many difficulties, vanquishing many monsters, and interacting with the gods. The religious basis seems to be a tolerant fusion of Buddhism, Taoism and Confucianism with elements taken from all three.

A final example also comes from the Far East – *Deep River (3)* is a novel by the Japanese writer Shusaku Endo. It follows the journey of four very different Japanese people to India amidst the turmoil of the assassination of Indira Gandhi by Sikh extremists. Each of them makes different discoveries about themselves by the sacred river Ganges. One is a widower seeking a possible reincarnation of his wife. A second is a former soldier who is haunted by things he has seen and experienced in wartime Burma. A third has a kind of mystical relationship with a bird he has owned and wants to visit a bird sanctuary. And the last comes seeking love and encounters a former lover who has been a Catholic priest for a time. They are four remarkably different people all feeling the need to make a pilgrimage which will influence their inner lives.

Throughout these literary examples, the greatest interest is in the interior journey of the protagonists into greater -awareness and maturity, the relationship between inner and outer landscapes. The temptations, the difficulties and the monsters encountered along the way are mythic or narrative conventions to dramatise the inner journey. That relationship between our outer and inner journeys with a focus very much on the significance of the latter is what is embraced by the metaphor of travelling east. How then might we reflect on inner journeys not only in myth, legend or epic narrative but in our own day to day experience?

The Franciscan priest and writer Richard Rohr (who himself makes extensive use of themes from the *Odyssey*) writes persuasively about the tasks of the two halves of life. (4) The tasks of the first half of life are primarily ego driven: developing education, a career, gathering possessions, finding success, establishing a sexual identity. All this is necessary work and is good as far as it goes. However alongside this we develop a shadow side: "Your shadow is what you refuse to see about yourself, and what you do not want others to see." (5) We repress those things and instead develop an idealised image of ourselves, the persona we allow others and ourselves to see. If a particular situation generates anger in us out of all proportion to the issue, then emotions from our shadow side are probably at the root of it (the response of some Christians to the issue of homosexuality might well be a good example of this). "The persona does not choose to see evil in itself, so it always disguises it as good. The shadow self invariably presents itself as something like prudence, common sense, justice – - – when it is actually manifesting fear, control, manipulation, or even vengeance." (6) The kind of religion that is produced is moralistic, keen to establish its merits and superiority to others.

Incidentally, I wonder whether the professionally religious – the clergy – are particularly vulnerable to the creation of a persona with which they feel they have to live. Even if they are not put up on a pedestal, the expectations of congregations about how a woman or man of God should live can be stultifying. At the very least this means the necessity of being nice to everyone all the time! Some seem to identify so closely with the clerical persona that it is impossible to get behind the mask. One wonders if they go to bed at night wearing a clerical collar. All this can get in the way of honest relationships and prevent the ordained themselves developing their inner lives in the most creative ways. I am puzzled as to what extent traditional relationships between clergy and laity are life enhancing and to what extent they are impoverishing.

This whole dynamic Rohr describes as the creation of the False Self. The False Self is not bad in itself but if we remain with it we have mistaken the part for the whole. We need to let it go at the right time as we begin the work of discovering more important truths about ourselves. This is the work of the second half of life, the discovery of the True Self. We are journeying eastwards and the tools of quietness, reflection and contemplation are needed far more than in the first half of life. On this journey we shall discover that we no longer need to define ourselves in opposition to others. Instead we can look at things we have in common. We no longer need to prove our superiority or want to punish others. Bolstering our egos is much less necessary. The focus is more on our inner experience. Our encounters with failure, disappointments and necessary suffering will often assist us in this exploration more than our successes and achievements -hence the description of this second half of life work as "falling upward." The dying to aspects of the Self in order that new things might come to life is a central part of the pattern of death and resurrection to be found throughout the universe. Dying we live.

"Your True Self is that part of you that knows who you are and whose you are, although largely unconsciously. Your False Self is just who you think you are." (7) Rohr variously identifies the True Self with the soul and the indwelling presence of the Spirit of God. The longing for the True Self at our heart and the longing for God are the same longing. The discovery of the True Self is at the same time the discovery of God. "Your True Self is who you are, and always have been in God, and at its core it is love itself. Love is both who you are and who you are still becoming." (8) This is the goal of our search for what is completely dependable and utterly reliable. We come to know that we are, in Rohr's memorable phrase, "held together by the glue of a universal love." (9)

The notion of mining provides the central metaphor in one of Rohr's recent books. In the second half of life a lot of debris has to be cleared out of the way so that we can get down to the "immortal diamond" which is the very centre of our life where we begin to discover that we live in God and God lives in us. "We each set out trying to create our own hand-cut and hand made diamond, but experienced pilgrims tell us that the diamond was first made by Another, and it is indeed drawing us forward into a brilliance that is now uniquely ours." (10) This is "Christ in you, the hope of glory." (11)

So journeying eastwards means reflecting on what aspects of this work in the second half of life have loomed large for me so far. I have begun to recognise some of the personas behind which I have attempted to construct my life: The Man Of God – - – The Scholar – - – The Social Animal – - -The Radical Theologian, and so on. All of them saying something about me but equally all of them completely inadequate as a description of who I am. As I wrote in the Downtown chapter, I have begun to see how a false perfectionism and its partner need always to be loved / liked have impacted on me. Later chapters will focus on some other areas that have come to prominence in recent years. For the moment I want to expand on two words that have increasingly assumed an importance for me: waiting and attentiveness.

I know rather a lot about waiting. I have to do quite a lot of it. I wait for assistance to get me up in the morning and to put me to bed at night. I wait for help with food and drink and getting to the toilet. My reaction to these enforced waits hovers between the poles of cheerful acceptance and resentful anger. But alongside this waiting because I have no choice something interesting is happening. I am learning how to wait in a new and positive way. "Sometimes I sit and think, and sometimes

I just sit" as a caption I saw years ago on a poster had it. That in itself has been something rather new for me. Like many ministers in the Reformation traditions, I have believed that it is faith not works which brings us freedom and then spent most of my working life dashing from one worthwhile activity to the next. But there is more to it than that. It feels as though in the silence, quite often beyond language or even conscious connected thoughts, I am waiting for something to be shown to me. It is not that waiting is a technique to prepare me for prayer. Rather, the waiting and the silence themselves are the praying. More about this when we travel Up North.

W H Vanstone argued that there are styles of waiting which are profound human experiences, like the lover who declares their feelings and then must wait for a response from the beloved. (12) We see how Jesus experienced this in the movement from action to passion. In his ministry he had been the focus for action, the main mover whether as preacher, teacher or healer. Now he must wait upon the decisions and behaviour of others: the High Priests, the Roman Governor, the soldiers. Yet in the weakness and helplessness of his waiting we discover profound truth no less than in his active ministry. Indeed, we give the events from Gethsemane to Calvary central importance for Christian faith. Perhaps as a person with disabilities, I am invited to reflect on the presence of God in those periods of waiting which feel negative and painful as well as in the more positive because chosen waiting times. That sounds fairly challenging! Yet Vanstone suggests also that there is a sense in which God waits for our response or perhaps more widely the response of all creation. God has poured out his love on his creation and now awaits the response (perhaps of wonder, love and praise) of the beloved. In so far as creation in its bondage fails to respond in that way and therefore fails to be its true self, so God experiences the pain of waiting.

The fruit of some of my waiting has been the beginning of a new attentiveness. I observe Henry, my daughter's black labrador, stretched out in the sunshine watching the world go by past the end of my driveway. I am struck powerfully both by his sheer aliveness and by how the workings of his mind and how he relates to the world around him are a complete mystery to me. Henry and I both watch a beetle make its way across the patio. As far as I can tell, the presence of both of us is equally a matter of complete indifference to it. Yet the three of us share a common quality of aliveness.

This paying attention to detail in the ordinary life around me is not something I have tried to cultivate before. Once the natural world would have had to take the form of a range of mountains or a dramatic seascape before I would take much notice. Now I am much more aware of the ordinary birds and flowers in my garden. It is obvious this is new because in the past, when two friends invited me on one of their birdwatching expeditions, my elder daughter who knows me well commented that she hoped I was taking a good novel along with me! I am still lamentably ignorant when it comes to identifying flora and fauna, but perhaps that doesn't necessarily matter too much? Indeed, the suggestion in a poem by Alastair Reid is that naming might actually sometimes be a drawback:

"Say the soft bird's name, but do not be surprised to see it fall / headlong, struck skyless, into its pigeonhole – / columba palumbus and you have it dead, / wedged, neat, unwinged in your head. – - –

The point is the seeing – the grace / beyond recognition, the ways / of the bird rising, unnamed, unknown, / beyond the range of language, beyond its noun. / Eyes open on growing, flying, happening, / and go on opening. Manifold, the world /

dawns on unrecognising, realising eyes. / Amazement is the thing. / Not love, but the astonishment of loving." (13)

I begin to understand that it is the paying attention, the seeing, which is the important thing. Only so do we begin to realise the intrinsic value of things. There is no need to rush off down a conventionally religious path and begin to talk about a sacramental world or something similar – as though the only purpose of the flower, the bird, the waterfall or the mountain was to point beyond itself to God. That feels like just one more type of utilitarianism – seeing things as means to an end. Yet it is the giving of attention that can foster a sense of wonder, and perhaps also there is no other way of learning to love people as well as things than by giving them proper attention. "The substance of love of our neighbour is an attentive way of looking." (Simone Weil) (14)

Barbara Glasson worked for a number of years as a minister in "pioneering communities" which are very much on the edge of conventional church. She uses the model of "coming out" from the experience of people discovering their sexual identity, survivors of abuse in early life and those wrestling with issues relating to disability or addiction in order to reflect on issues affecting both the Church and wider culture as a whole. What seems particularly interesting from the perspective of my reflection is the similarity in much of the language that she uses:

"Solidarity with those within the coming-out process is one of the most profound transformative experiences. It involves a very deep attentiveness to those things that are beyond words, to the inner processes of the emergent self and to the paradoxical experiences that form layer upon layer in the creation of the new person. Giving attention to another, to the inner commotion of "I am not" within the deepest silence of acknowledged experience is a deeply challenging task. – - – I want to acknowledge – - – a theology of mess if you like in which we can enter into the depths of unknowing in order to find the truth about self within the context of faith." (15)

This paying attention, this learning to look and see, seems a very different thing than a rather sentimental conventional piety. Indeed it feels more like a frequently challenging art to learn on the road to discovering how things and people might be loved in their often hugely difficult difference. Willy Loman in Arthur Miller's play *Death of a Salesman is* a far from attractive character but late on in the play his wife says of him:

"He is not the finest character that ever lived. But he is a human being, and a terrible thing is happening to him. So attention must be paid. He is not to be allowed to fall into his grave like an old dog. Attention, attention must finally be paid to such a person." (16)

Having said all that, I read somewhere that one of the root meanings of the word "religion" may be "to pay attention." Perhaps a key dynamic of a religious life is that learning to pay attention through which we learn how to love. Moreover, the idea of "the numinous" which we usually associate with a sense of awe and mystery when encountering the divine comes in part from the Latin nuo meaning "I nod." The thing or person that we see nods at us as though to say, I am inviting your undivided attention in this moment. "Everything beckons to us to perceive it." (Rilke) It is not that the active observer gazes at the passive object. Instead that which I perceive is given to me, freely, and a current of recognition flows between us – in Gerard Manley Hopkins' famous line, "the world is charged with the grandeur of God." Michael Mayne describes the result of this as "the transfigured commonplace." This can frequently feel quite ordinary and everyday but sometimes has a remarkable power to it, as reflected in a poem by Sylvia Plath: "A certain minor light may still / Leap incandescent / Out of kitchen table or chair / As if a celestial burning took / Possession of the most obtuse objects now and then – / Thus hallowing an interval / Otherwise inconsequent / By bestowing largesse, honour, / One might say love." (17) What does this echo other than the story of Moses at the burning bush?

Sallie McFague splendidly summarises this process that I have begun to explore and tried to explain:

"I have learned that the closer attention I pay to whatever piece of the world is before me – the more I know about it, the more open I am to its presence, the closer I look at it or listen to it or touch it or smell it – the more amazed I am by it. It is not that I "see God in it" in any direct or general way, rather, it is the specialness, the difference, the intricacy of each creature, event or aspect of nature that calls forth wonder." (18)

It might be objected that all this sounds rather introverted and indeed self-indulgent. This is certainly a danger yet many witnesses in the Christian tradition suggest that it can generate a greater concern, a more sensitive awareness towards those who are disadvantaged, excluded or oppressed. For many years the Taizé Community has been encouraging the bringing together of "struggle and contemplation." I have recently gained tremendously through reading the autobiography of the American Christian Sara Miles. (19) An investigative journalist and left-wing activist, she had thoroughly rejected the evangelical religion of her parents. Yet through an almost mystical encounter with the celebration of the Eucharist, she was led into founding a food kitchen which eventually had a large number of bases feeding hundreds of needy people across San Francisco. And if we go back to the most basic Christian witness of all, we can recall that in the parable of Jesus the failure of the rich man was in part that he paid no attention, did not even notice, Lazarus, the beggar at his gate. (20)

This silence and attentiveness, this waiting and looking, this moving beyond conscious thought and language, all seem to me to be part of that second half of life task of discovering the True Self. The journey Up North will explore some particular dimensions of this before I attempt to pull together some of these travelling insights.

(1) Robert Macfarlane: Mountains Of the Mind (Granta 2003 paperback edition 2008)

(2) Kosuke Koyama: 3 Mile an Hour God (SCM 1979)

(3) Shusaku Endo: Deep River (Sceptre new addition 1995)

(4) Richard Rohr: Falling Upward (Jossey-Bass 2011)

(5) Falling Upward.

(6) Falling Upward.

(7) Richard Rohr: Immortal Diamond (SPCK 2013)

(8) Immortal Diamond

(9) Immortal Diamond

(10) Immortal Diamond

(11) Colossians 1: 27

(12) W H Vanstone: The Stature of Waiting (Darton, Longman and Todd 1982)

(13) Alistair Reid from "Growing, Flying, Happening." Quoted in Michael Mayne: This Sunrise of Wonder, (1995 new edition Darton, Longman and Todd 2008)

(14) Quoted in This Sunrise of Wonder.

(15) Barbara Glasson: The Exuberant Church (Darton, Longman and Todd 2011)

(16) Quoted in This Sunrise of Wonder.

(17) Sylvia Plath from "Black Rook in Rainy Weather." Quoted in This Sunrise of Wonder.

(18) Sallie McFague: The Body of God An Ecological Theology (SCM 1993)

(19) Sara Miles: Take This Bread (Canterbury Press 2012)

(20) Luke 16: 19-31

VI
Up North

Broadly speaking, if you want to discover harsher landscapes in Britain you travel (with apologies to the Brecon Beacons and Snowdonia) north to the Pennines, Cumbria or the Scottish Highlands. The experts tell us that there is no such thing as proper wilderness country in Great Britain. However, picking your way down from the summit of Great Gable in thick mist and driving November rain can feel quite wild enough – this on a day when I was introducing a friend to the delights of Lake District fell walking for the first time! Our mountainous areas may be modest in height but they still deserve caution and respect: every year brings fatalities and injuries on the hills. The reports of the mountain rescue services catalogue a variety of inexperience, unsuitable equipment and sheer bad luck. Even Wainwright, writing about being lost on his favourite fell Haystacks, offers the interesting advice that the only thing a novice can do in such circumstances is to "kneel down and pray for deliverance."

It is relatively recently that mountainous areas have been seen as attractive playgrounds where an element of danger is part of the attraction. For hundreds of years they were seen as hostile, to be avoided on all possible occasions, the dwelling place of evil forces. Early travellers across the Alpine passes sometimes wore blindfolds in case they were completely overwhelmed by the sight of the towering crags around them. The outlook which considered wild places to be attractive places didn't really develop until the eighteenth century. It was then that the first guidebooks to areas like the Lake District began to gain popularity. The philosophical notion of "The Sublime" saw a combination of delight and terror experienced from a position of safety as the appropriate reaction to mountain views. Mountains were not seen as beautiful (a concept applied more frequently to pastoral, often man-made landscapes) so much as sublime. Wild places began to be sought out rather than avoided, or at least "Picturesque" views of crags, hillsides and waterfalls were identified and visitors were advised of the best "stations" from which they could be admired.

The whole Romantic movement, rooted in the eighteenth century but coming to full flower in the first half of the nineteenth, gave a tremendous impetus to this new way of looking, a perspective of which we are the inheritors. This was a wide ranging revolution with enormous impact on both literature and the visual arts. It was reflected in a practical way by Wordsworth tramping tens of thousands of miles up hill and down dale and Coleridge ignoring safety and common sense whilst climbing on Scafell. Even Keats, who was far from being a great climber, apparently used to imagine mountaintop scenery as a way to combat his insomnia.

Present-day attitudes would have been incomprehensible to people only two or three hundred years ago. Daniel Defoe produced the account of his tour around Britain in the 1720s:

"Defoe had no time for mountains; – - – they had "a kind of unhospitable terror in them." For him the hills of Cumberland and Westmorland had no redeeming features; they had no rich pleasant valleys like the Alps, no lead mines like the Peak District, no coal pits like the hills around Halifax and no gold like the Andes. They were "all barren and wild, of no use or advantage either to man or beast." For Defoe there was nothing spiritually uplifting or aesthetically pleasing about mountain scenery." (1)

Compare this to our own day with mountains being "automatically venerated forms of landscape, images of which permeate an urbanised Western culture increasingly hungry for even second-hand experiences of wildness and wilderness." (2) Even a few moments' thought while resting against the summit cairn is enough to remind the climber that there is more here than just being on top of the world looking down on creation. A new perspective is gained of both time and space: the immense aeons of time which have gone into forming the mountains and the views of ranges of hills stretching away to the horizon whilst the sky seems to go on forever. What amounts to a feeling of vertigo is produced by a mixture of wonder with a sense of human insignificance.

It becomes obvious that we do not view landscapes objectively in themselves. We bring to our viewing perceptions inherited from our culture which has taught us to see in particular ways. In other words we bring interpretation into the situation, usually unconsciously. I had always assumed that exploring mountainous country was the prerogative of experts and superfit heroes. Then sometime in 1980 I found myself in a bookshop in Cumbria and came across Wainwright's guidebooks. (3) Glancing at them produced something of an epiphany moment for me. It appeared that this mountain walking was something even I could tackle! Granted that Helvellyn was not K2, this looked as though it could be a whole new area of modest adventuring for me. By request my next birthday produced the gift of the pictorial guides and so began an interest, an enthusiasm, a minor obsession which was to take up a big part of my leisure time for the next dozen years or so. When there were no holidays with opportunities to be on the tops, I would be studying potential new routes as my bedtime reading.

So now I have a host of mountain memories: pleasant uneventful days, wet and rather miserable days, spectacular days.

I remember climbing Skiddaw up the tourist track above Keswick. It is quite a long slog and on this occasion a thick grey mist obscured everything apart from a few yards before and behind. Then within a hundred feet or so of the summit I came out above the cloud into a new world of bright sunshine. The whole of the Lake District as far as the eye could see was covered in what can only be described as the clichéd cotton wool. Only the very highest peaks – the Scafells, Helvellyn, Great Gable – peeked out above all this billowing sea of whiteness. It was my only, and unforgettable, experience of that kind of cloud inversion. The seventeenth century diarist John Evelyn had a similar experience which he described with typically English restraint: "This was I must acknowledge one of the most pleasant, new and altogether surprising objects that in my life I had ever beheld."

A call of the wild seems to be heard by many people although not, incidentally, by my late father-in-law who could never see the point of slogging up hillsides. His response to an enthusiasm about the views from the summits was simply to say that there were plenty of excellent views to be had at sea level. However, the wilderness provides opportunities for many people to match themselves in ways appropriate to their abilities. At the extremes it produces heroic figures of exploration, whether of the polar ice caps, the Himalayas or the desert. Heroism whether tragic or triumphant stirs the imagination of lesser mortals who learn about Shackleton and Scott, Lawrence of Arabia or Mallory and Hillary. More broadly, David Jasper in his erudite work examines an eclectic mixture of philosophers, travellers, filmmakers and theologians who have been influenced by "the sacred desert."

There is of course a very long tradition of associating both mountains and deserts with aspects of the religious life, whether in actuality or their use as metaphors. Images of desert, cloud and mountain have been "used on the one hand to question the overconfidence in words that sometimes characterises the theological enterprise, and on the other hand to suggest metaphorically the deepest, virtually indescribable, human experiences of pain and joy." (4) In the Judaeo-Christian tradition the archetypal story is that of Moses on Mount Sinai, together with the time spent both by the people of Israel and by Jesus himself in the wilderness. Having received a divine call at the burning bush in the wilderness, it is in the midst of the cloud and darkness at Sinai that Moses encounters God and where he is allowed to glimpse God's back but not his face from his position in a cleft in the rock. (5) At the beginning of his public ministry Jesus is driven – the Greek word used in Mark's Gospel literally means "thrown out" – to the wilderness by the Spirit of God, there to confront his own demons. (6)

One of the influential themes going back in Christian tradition at least as far as the early fourth century monks in the deserts of Egypt and Syria is known as apophatic ("beyond images") theology or sometimes the via negativa, the way of negation. It stresses the inability of the mind to grasp the reality of God. Indeed God is not an object that can be grasped or understood like other objects. We know the reality of the divine only in the silence which is beyond thoughts or experience. "The true knowledge and vision of God consists in this – in seeing that He is invisible, because what we seek lies beyond all knowledge, being wholly separated by the darkness of incomprehensibility." (7) Amidst this darkness and silence, this awareness of the absence of God, new discoveries of loving and being loved can be made, as the contemplative tradition explores.

"What the desert teaches is a radical letting go of the thinking-experiencing-managing self, so as to be content with God alone, a God without adjectives, without comforting signs of presence so that at last one learns truly to delight in nothing – - – The meaning of the mystery is no longer an anxious concern of those who have been to the desert. Naming implies a control that the wilderness no longer allows." (8)

This can be a tough journey. It recognises the inadequacy of all our religious language in sharp distinction to what E M Forster described as "poor, talkative little Christianity." It embraces a fierce and demanding approach which is a long way removed from the feel good nature of much contemporary spirituality. It strips bare the false claims of our egos and our anxious need for religious experiences. It invites us to an indifference to (or perhaps detachment from) those things that do not really matter in order to focus on those things which do. "Teach us to care and not to care." (9) This is mirrored in the external wilderness landscape where a fierce beauty is also a reminder of its indifference to the needs of human beings. The shattered scree slopes will continue to tumble into Wastwater whether anyone observes them or not; they are indifferent to whether I or anyone else lives or dies. Our complacent notion that the world is there solely for our benefit is thoroughly undermined. Some even posit a recognition of the indifference of God out of which a new experience of divine love may emerge:

"In the vast resources of divine disinterest a freedom and a joy that is missing in much of contemporary pop theology – - – I really don't want a God who is solicitous of my every need, fawning for my attention, eager for nothing in the world so much as the fulfilment of my self potential. One of the scourges of our age is that all our deities are housebroken and eminently companionable. Far from demanding anything, they ask only how they can more meaningfully enhance the lives of those they serve." (10)

Moreover, the wilderness experience is far from being a privatised concern between the individual and the divine. The early monks, living in the desert on the edge of things, discovered a new attentiveness to the world around them and a new perspective on the society of the towns and cities. People travelled into the desert to seek their wisdom and advice as they had a few centuries previously when people flocked from the towns into the wilderness to listen to the uncompromising preaching of John the Baptist. Their new mode of Christian living in itself was a critique of their contemporary church and its accommodations with the outlook and priorities of wider society.

I hear echoes for the contemporary Western Church which is increasingly finding itself living at the margins. This seems to be true whether the situation is described as post-modern, post-Christendom or even post-Christian. There does not appear to be any end to the long process whereby Christian values and assumptions, once taken for granted as the air that everyone breathed, have become the outlook of a relatively small minority. The institutional church finds its new position very frequently at the edge of things a difficult one to which to adjust. However, some interpreters of the situation suggest that life at the margins gives new opportunities to relate to the wider society in new ways. On the margins might be a suitable place from which to offer a prophetic critique of the assumptions and priorities holding sway nearer the centre. Recent examples have included church reports critical of the way in which government and others misrepresent issues of poverty, a challenging of many of the assumptions behind welfare reforms and the attack by none other than the Archbishop of

Canterbury on the ethics of payday loan companies. Perhaps it becomes more possible too for the church to pay attention to the voices of others who are marginalised. (11)

Darkness, silence, absence, emptiness, love born when the anxious concerns of the ego are stripped away – these are recurring themes in the Christian tradition. We find them in the anonymous fourteenth century work *The Cloud of Unknowing*, in the Spanish mystics St Teresa of Avila and St John of the Cross, in the writings of Thomas Merton. Some have suggested that there is a new interest in these ancient ways in our post-modern context. "Modernity has failed to understand anything about the desert except as a place to be wearily traversed by one or two brave souls in the service of Empire, and has absorbed the mystic path into its positivisms though, miraculously, the desert wind is again blowing in the unlikely wastes of post-modernity." (12) Perhaps those of us in the Protestant traditions are particularly in need of their insights, belonging as we do to "one of the noisiest forms of Christianity – the least attentive to the silence of God in Christian history." (13) Yet I rather think you would have to search diligently to uncover evidence of that interest. Much more frequently we resemble the description attributed to the Methodist scholar Gordon Rupp: we are like an old-fashioned swimming baths where most of the noise is made by those splashing about in the shallow end. This feels rather more typical of much contemporary Christianity than the kind of experience described by the Welsh priest and poet RS Thomas: "Why no! I never thought other than / That God is that great absence / In our lives, the empty silence / Within, the place where we go / Seeking, not in hope to / Arrive or find." (14)

Wilderness imagery continues to resonate powerfully in wider contemporary culture. The former Monty Python member

Michael Palin felt its power whilst making his travel documentary about the Sahara: "This is landscape reduced to its barest essentials, a rippling, rolling, shadeless surface purged of every living. The immense emptiness quietens everyone. Progress is slow and steady, although such is the lack of distinctive landmarks it sometimes feels as if we are walking on the spot." (15)

In unlikely fashion we move from Palin to TS Eliot; it was the desert which provided Eliot with one of the metaphors to light up the fragility of relationships and language itself in the years following 1918: there we find "a heap of broken images where the sun beats / and the dead tree gives no shelter." (16) The inadequacy of language, the movement towards silence and the necessity of stillness and waiting are recurring themes in his poetry.

Wilderness landscape not just as a backdrop but as a vital influence on the narrative continues to be important in a variety of media. It is there in a novel such as Jim Crace's *Quarantine* with its imaginative weaving together of the Biblical account of Jesus' temptations and a group of travellers who have arrived in the Judaean desert for a variety of reasons:

"Jesus – - -had seen the footprints of the little group of travellers who had preceded him, deviating from the camel trail. He could have followed them and passed his quarantine in company, tucked into the folds of clay, amongst the poppies, and exposed to nothing worse than forty days of boredom and discomfort. But Jesus had a harsher challenge for himself. Quite what it was he didn't know. He only understood that he should choose a way that was more punishing. The worse it was, the better it would be. That, surely, was the purpose of the wilderness. He knew the scriptures and the stories of the prophets. Triumph over hardship was their proof of holiness." (17)

The fierce and harsh beauty of the North African desert is more a protagonist than simply a background to the novel / film *The English Patient (18)*, bringing the lovers together and tearing them apart in a story of passion and tragedy. It is there too in another Oscar-winning film *No Country For Old Men* (19) based on the novel by Cormac McCarthy where the wild country of the Texas desert is a place of casual brutality and sometimes psychotic savagery by those who live around it. The opening scenes of the movie in particular show dramatic images of the beauty and harshness of the desert landscape. The fourth century desert fathers and mothers might discover some themes they were familiar with in this poem by the American poet, artist and traveller Jan Haas:

"I walked off the highway, / back behind the beer bottle line, / among the rabbit tracks and the Sidewinder trails / back in the winter sand – barefoot / looking for miles, beyond eternity / and the grey hills bronzed by the setting sun, / in the wind and the silence, wishing we were gone / and our shacks had fallen into ruin / so our grandchildren could hear tales / of the settlers who tried to make it here / when the land was still untamed / and who left / because they didn't want to make a garden / out of the grandeur of God's desert / or an oasis out of the sand." (20)

Paradoxically, in some ways, in the midst of our urban existence, the wilderness comes to us with fresh immediacy. Thanks to the technological brilliance of modern equipment and the remarkable attentiveness and patience of wildlife photographers, I can swoop over the African Sahara or the

Australian outback and moments later be actually inside the burrow of a strange desert dwelling rodent. In much harsher mode, the deserts of Iraq, Libya and Syria and the mountainous regions of Afghanistan and Pakistan are rarely far from the news. The wilderness silence is broken by the scream of jet fighters, the clatter of helicopters and the roar of heavy artillery. Unmanned drones bring death from the skies with terrifying suddenness. Equally suddenly improvised explosive devices hidden in the sand produce carnage. Weapons of mass destruction prove to be as substantial as a desert mirage. The harshness of the wilderness has new victims in the dead and bereaved, the physically maimed and those whose mental and emotional traumas will last a lifetime. The story of Western empire builders coming to grief amidst the mountains and deserts is a lengthy one. As long ago as the fifth century BC the Greek historian Herodotus recounted the legend of an army in Libya which was dispatched to defeat the storm god of the desert only to disappear without trace (the works of Herodotus including this tale are used in the novel and film based on it *The English Patient*). Yet millennia later, Western hubris codenamed the first Gulf war campaign Operation Desert Storm.

My mountain walking days are behind me. I would need a mountain rescue team to get me over the first stile! The nearest I have come to the physicality of desert terrain is when I have struggled through the sand dunes carrying the enormous amount of equipment required for a family day out on the beach. Yet the spirituality associated with the wilderness fascinates me more and more.

"The desert as metaphor is that uncharted terrain beyond the edges of the seemingly secure and structured world in which we take such confidence, a world of affluence and order we cannot imagine ever ending. Yet it does. And the point where the world begins to crack, where brokenness and disorientation suddenly overtake us, then we step into the wide, silent plains of a desert we had never known existed. – - – Only there does love reveal itself in unaccountable wonder." (21)

I need the words of the traveller and the poet, the images of the filmmaker and photographer and the reflections of the theologian to stimulate my imagination in relation to the exterior landscapes of mountain and desert. And so they continue to have their impact on the interior landscape of my Christian understanding and discipleship. The poet Robert Frost feels a sense of loneliness contemplating a snowy landscape and the night sky but then concludes: "They cannot scare me with their empty spaces / Between stars – on stars where no human race is. / I have it in me so much nearer home / To scare myself with my own desert places." (22) Perhaps the new world into which I have been introduced by disability is a wilderness world of penetrating questions, challenges and opportunities. Where accepted patterns, assumed identity and expectations are all needing review. Part of the via negativa is the honest confronting of brokenness and weakness, a new narrative which contradicts the cultural norm of defining human value in terms of productivity and social capital. Part of its promise is that through that process might emerge a new experience of loving which is the only way in which God can be known. The hope that in the waiting and the silence a word of love might be heard. Is this the "Sound of sheer silence" which Elijah heard in the desert? (23) Is this what the heart yearns for most?

(1) Ian Thompson: The English Lakes A History (Bloomsbury, 2010)

(2) Robert Macfarlane: Mountains Of the Mind (Granta 2003 paperback edition 2008)

(3) Alfred Wainwright: A Pictorial Guide to the Lakeland Fells (seven volumes 1952-1966)

(4) Belden G Lane: The Solace Of Fierce Landscapes (Oxford University Press, 1998)

(5) Exodus 3: 1ff, 24:15ff, 33: 17ff

(6) Mark 1: 12

(7) Gregory of Nyssa (c 335 – c 395CE)

(8) The Solace Of Fierce Landscapes.

(9) TS Eliot from "Ash Wednesday" in Collected Poems 1909-1962 (Faber and Faber 1963)

(10) The Solace Of Fierce Landscapes.

(11) I pursued some of this thinking at greater length in Disabled Church?

(12) David Jasper: The Sacred Desert Religion, Literature, Art and Culture (Blackwell 2004)

(13) Diarmaid MacCulloch: Silence A Christian History (Penguin 2013)

(14) Quoted in The Sacred Desert.

(15) Michael Palin: Sahara (Weidenfeld and Nicholson 2010)

(16) TS Eliot from "The Wasteland" in Collected Poems 1909-1962 (Faber and Faber 1963)

(17) Jim Crace: Quarantine (Viking 1997)

(18) Michael Ondaatje: The English Patient (Bloomsbury 1992)

(19) Cormack McCarthy: No Country For Old Men (Picador 2005)

(20) From Jan Haag: "Arizona Desert" accessed at www.janhaag.com

(21) The Solace Of Fierce Landscapes.

(22) Robert Frost: "Desert Places" in Selected Poems (Penguin, 1953)

(23) I Kings 19:12

VII
Travelling
Companions

A former colleague once spoke witheringly to me about a particular style of spirituality which he described as "Jesus and me." The sort of question at the centre of this approach might be: What has Jesus done for me this week? How have I been blessed in the last month? This might be something of a caricature but it makes the point. Too much Christianity seems to think that the be all and end all of Christian living is my individual relationship with the Lord. One of the ways to avoid that trap, it seems to me, is to remind ourselves regularly of the variety of people who have been our travelling companions on the Christian way. So here is a brief excursion on which to see snapshots of some of those who have accompanied, influenced or taught me in the things of Christ. To avoid self-consciousness or embarrassment to anyone, I am limiting myself to some of those who have died, aware of course that their numbers could be greatly increased by others who are still amongst the living.

So here is Edna Proctor, not a biological parent but definitely a mother figure to "her " young people in the youth fellowship she runs, caring deeply and fussing over her charges; next to Edna her husband James, retired primary headteacher, sucking laconically on his pipe and shaking his head in mild bemusement at the antics of adolescents. Here are Herbert and Annie Revell, people of transparent goodness and innocence which through their long life together has never been spoiled by the frequently perplexing world which they have observed and experienced. Here are Lewis and Irene Stockdale, Methodists to the core of their being, large people squeezing themselves into their Reliant Robin with a pile of catering equipment for the latest church event; offering open house hospitality to a young bachelor minister to drop in any time he felt like a meal or some conversation.

Here is Ethel Lily, speaking publicly in church for the first time when she was well over 80, describing how life for a long time had felt as though it had a dark cloud hovering over it and how one day as she stood at her sink and sang the words of "Jesu, lover of my soul" it felt as though that cloud finally began to lift. Here is Nelly Taafe, amputee with a wicked sense of humour, allowing herself to be carried unceremoniously up the steps in her wheelchair so that she could attend evening service. Here is Anne Cotterill, recently widowed, leaving her home one Sunday morning and finding herself attending her local Methodist church for the first time; it was the beginning of remarkable ministry in which she was courier for the church community transport scheme, helping to bring the semi-housebound to meals and midweek meetings in all weathers; later she became a leader of midweek worship and, much to her constant amazement, a Church Steward. Here is Nelly Allen, retired Baptist deaconess, very kindly in general conversation but extremely feisty in matters religious especially when it came to correct or incorrect doctrines – love the Minister but hate his theological standpoints!

Here is Fred Jones, gifted artist but completely self-effacing, the epitome of a modest, gentle man for whom undertaking a piece of down-to-earth service without thought of praise or even acknowledgement just came naturally; several of his watercolours hang in my home, generous gifts representing a generous man. Here is Monica Bowles, tragically bereaved by traffic accident of her husband and one of her sons; showing immense courage and resilience and retaining a lovely, warm interest in others; finding strength for her faith in the community of her local village chapel, a building which had a key place in both her affection and her Christian living. Here is David Cleland, bringing his incisive mind and organisational skills to the world of education and the work of a lay preacher; bringing a generosity of spirit and care for local ministers together with a combination of diplomacy and determination to the task of Methodist Circuit Steward (a senior Methodist lay person). Here is Wyn Knight, widowed after a long marriage to a husband who was a committed Marxist and socialist; much to her surprise, finding herself at home late in life in her local church; putting the local Conservative MP and TV celebrity in his place without any difficulty. Here is Jean Smeatham, a model of kindness, graciousness and good humour; nothing like the caricature of a church organist, we shared many chuckles about the vagaries of wedding parties.

Some of the Superintendent ministers with whom I have worked. Here is Alex Heyes, his opening prayers when leading worship were so long that a teenager on the back row who had had a late Saturday night could fall asleep in them without waiting for the sermon; but to talk to him one-to-one was to find aspects of Jesus really coming alive. Here is Gordon Simmonds, who showed me the value in a combination of liturgical worship and thoughtful preaching. Here is Greg Carter, superintendent when I had my first appointment as a probationer minister; he had found ways to be at home in his life and ministry; the day before my first Sunday appointments, he prayed with me in the church and tears ran down his face as he remembered the beginning of his own ministry forty or so years before. Other ministers who have continued to support me even when I have neglected them. And here is Robert Hey who took me under his wing just before and in the early stages of my ministerial training; thrilled to bits to have been accepted as one of Mr Wesley's itinerant preachers; absolutely committed to a traditional ministry of Word and Sacrament; dead far too young of a degenerative lung condition.

As the writer of the Letter to the Hebrews put it, there just isn't time to mention everyone. (1) The more I wander back haphazardly over the years, the more faces emerge again into the conscious part of my mind. They are all members of my communion of saints. Nothing is more sure about this piece of my work than that after it is finished I shall regret having missed out some names. We have been "Pilgrims on a journey and companions on the road." We have been "here to help each other walk the mile and bear the load." (2) I remember once again that the root meaning of companions is "those who break bread together."

I am familiar with the instruction of Jesus that his followers should travel light. (3) Familiar but no good at all at actually keeping to it. So I shall need a large suitcase or rucksack into which will go all sorts of other friends for the journey.

I am not going to be a castaway on a desert island, instructed that I must be very limited in my choices. So there will be some favourite CDs by those whose music has accompanied me since teenage years: Leonard Cohen, Joni Mitchell, Paul Simon, Beach Boys, Motown. The compilation album of "Songs of the Century" (chosen by Radio Two listeners, illustrating how irredeemably middle of the road I am) which helped to keep me sane during a lengthy spell in hospital and which was played through my headphones on the afternoon when it was first suggested that progressive MS was the likely cause of the symptoms I was experiencing. There will definitely have to be a selection of hymns – from Charles Wesley to John Bell but managing to live without many of the Victorian efforts which remains so popular with many congregations. And definitely no Moody and Sankey! But it would be a major mistake to go without Mozart's Clarinet Concerto and some Beethoven – perhaps a couple of Violin Romances and the Emperor Concerto. There will also need to be some representative "sacred" music, excerpts from The Messiah and a classical setting of the Mass perhaps. Oh and "Jesu, joy of man's desiring."

There needs to be food for the eyes as well as the ears of course. So in go a good number of photographs either in old-fashioned albums or equally old-fashioned slides – nothing in digital format unless I can squeeze a laptop in somewhere. From family shots of children growing up to maiden great aunts in their earlier existence as 1920s flappers. Plus some DVDs of films that have made a huge impact on me, ones that have stunned me into silence, left me drained or stopped me in my tracks: *Oh! What A Lovely War, One Flew Over The Cuckoo's Nest, Mississippi Burning, Philadel*phia. And perhaps just one all-time favourite for its humour: *Butch Cassidy And The Sundance Kid.*

I will naturally have the Bible and the Collected Works of Shakespeare. And the "Wainwrights" of course. Then a selection of the contemporary novels which have had more than usual impact on me. There may be some delay whilst I try and choose between works by: Ian McEwan, Marilynne Robinson, Jane Smiley, Khaled Hosseini, Susan Hill, Barbara Kingsolver, Niall Williams, Sebastian Barry, Pat Barker, Philip Roth, Kiran Desai, Sebastian Faulks, Penelope Lively, Arundhati Roy etc etc. The preacher at the service to mark my retirement commented that I got all my theology out of novels, and there was more than a grain of truth in what he said! And poetry? Probably TS Eliot should go in the case – I have long felt an affinity with Prufrock, and perhaps one day I will be able to work out what The *Wasteland* and *Four Quartets* are really all about.

Last but of course not least, a brief catalogue of some of the work that has provided theological highlights for me.

I arrived on the theological scene too late to experience the furore around John Robinson's *Honest to God.* (4) However I did read the work of Harvey Cox and others who were attempting to make some theological sense of the secularisation process. With hindsight, developments were much more varied and nuanced than they imagined but I do think that some of the work from the 60s and early 70s about the nature of the servant Church could do with being revisited sometimes. And I still nod agreement with the pithy saying attributed to Cox: "If God read Time magazine, he would read the religious section last."

University life and ministerial training of course involved wrestling with some of the twentieth century theological greats. I was helped a great deal in this by a book entitled *The Question of God.* (5) I have rarely seen this book mentioned anywhere but it provided informative introductions to Barth, Tillich et al. Ideal for the undergraduate! Mind you, theology tutorials were never as embarrassing as English literature tutorials when it became clear that some students had only managed to read half the set text of some huge nineteenth century novel. Attempting to analyse the motivation of a character who doesn't appear until chapter 25 when you have only read as far as chapter 15 is an interesting exercise!

My blinkered understanding of the work of the Holy Spirit was opened up considerably when I read John V Taylor's *The Go Between God (6)* especially the early chapters on how the Spirit acts as a go-between in relationships between people and between a person and an object of beauty. I took the book down from my shelf again recently after I was invited to preach at a city centre church which was hosting a major Christian art exhibition and found its insights still spoke to me. As indeed does the slightly later work of W H Vanstone (7).

I have found wrestling to try and understand the relationship between cross and empty tomb to be a recurring theme for me, and Vanstone's exploration of the tragic and triumphant possibilities of love has always struck a chord. The poem which formed the final page of his book is now sung as a hymn (given the seal of approval by inclusion in the latest Methodist hymn book) with a theme of the open and hidden dimensions of loving which continues to resonate with me.

It is surely a shame when too rigid a boundary is placed between the areas of theology and spirituality. At least much of the work which I have found most helpful has managed to build bridges between those two areas. But amongst those whose writing would, I guess, be categorised as spirituality I would mention first of all Neville Ward. (8) A book by a Methodist minister about the rosary! Although I rarely made use of that method of praying, Ward's exploration of the various Joyful, Sorrowful and Glorious Mysteries was very stimulating. And others? Harry Williams (9), Alan Ecclestone (10), Kenneth Leech (11), Sheila Cassidy (12) all come to mind. What seems frequently to unite these authors is a breadth and depth of humanity unfettered by too much narrowly religious concern.

I first became properly aware of the field of "disability theology" through the writing of Nancy Eiesland. (13) Her writing is part of a new emphasis which goes further than the contemporary interest in self -giving and vulnerability as key aspects of a loving God:

"How can God be both omnipotent and disabled? The question is based on a false premise. We have too often based our notion of God's power on our human notions of power and success magnified to the nth degree. The crucified and risen Christ, the icon who bears the marks of disability, contradicts this. God's power is always the power of love which is suffering and vulnerable yet always too unquenched and undefeated. Not outside creation as an all-powerful deus ex machina but at the heart of it as the prompting power of love, as process theology expresses it, always attracting into a new future. Bearing the marks of disability is not a temporary experience which God went through in Christ but something which is an essential aspect of God's fundamental nature of love." (14)

It could reasonably be objected that the theological heavy-weights with whom I wrestled as a theology student – Bultmann, Pannenberg, Moltmann – are conspicuous by their absence from my list. I am sure I have absorbed insights from all of them, but my list is more about those who have really grabbed me and moved me on in my discipleship as well as my understanding. Perhaps the best religious writing moves both head and heart?

Notwithstanding the lack of heavy theological tomes, it is a good thing there are no flights involved on my journeys because I would be in danger of exceeding my baggage allowance! However, there is just one corner left and in it will go one more DVD. It will feature the Ashes heroics of Botham and Flintoff. The winning extra time goal by Ryan Giggs in the 1999 FA Cup semi-final replay against Arsenal. And I can't possibly go without the British gold medal winners at London 2012. ––––––

(1) Hebrews 11: 32

(2) Richard Gillard: "Brother, sister, let me serve you."

(3) Matthew 10: 9

(4) John A T Robinson: Honest to God (SCM 1963)

(5) Heinz Zahrnt: The Question of God (Collins 1969)

(6) John V Taylor: The Go-Between God (SCM 1972)

(7) W H Vanstone: Love's Endeavour Love's Expense (Darton Longman and Todd 1977)

(8) J Neville Ward: Five for Sorrow Ten For Joy (Epworth 1971), Friday Afternoon (Epworth 1976)

(9) Harry Williams: True Wilderness (Pelican 1968), True Resurrection (Mitchell Beazley 1972), Tensions (Mitchell Beazley 1976), The Joy of God (Mitchell Beazley 1979)

(10) Alan Ecclestone: Yes to God (Darton, Longman and Todd 1975)

(11) Kenneth Leech: True Prayer (Sheldon Press 1980)

(12) Sheila Cassidy: Sharing the Darkness (Darton, Longman and Todd 1988), Good Friday People (Darton, Longman and Todd 1991)

(13) Nancy Eiesland: The Disabled God Towards A Liberatory Theology Of Disability (Abingdon Press 1994)

(14) Graham Evans: Disabled Church? (Church in the Marketplace Publications 2010)

VIII
Blue Highways

A shelf full of travel books about the USA testifies to my enjoyment of that genre and my fascination with the United States. Some of them are light-hearted travelogues such as grouping together cities with a link to particular songs, from Chicago to Tulsa. Others are much more reflective. Amongst the latter is *Blue Highways* by William Least Heat-Moon. (1) In it the author undertakes a long circular journey by Camper Van around the States. He follows a rather meandering course of back roads and byways: the book's title is derived from the fact that on old maps the freeways were marked in red whilst what in Britain would be called minor roads were coloured blue.

This feels like another helpful metaphor for my Christian journey. For a long time it has not felt as though I was motoring down a freeway. Instead, like travelling down a country road, I have been frequently surprised by what has appeared around the next bend and from time to time the way has turned out to be a dead end. So I want to attempt a summary of where the blue highways have taken me so far.

I recall one late June evening standing on the summit of one of the more modest Lakeland fells. Not a soul to be seen in any direction, the sunlight highlighting features on the higher summits and the sheep casting long shadows across the grass. In a way that was stimulated by the beauty around me but went beyond it, I experienced a powerful feeling of harmony and wholeness, a sense of belonging to creation. Fast forward to a rather different scenario. Laid aside with a bout of flu, I lay in bed listening to Desert Island Discs. The guest, whose identity I no longer recall, gave the opinion that his next choice was "the most profound piece of music ever written." Knowing nothing or virtually nothing about classical music I gave a snort of derision – and then listened for the first time to the slow movement from Mozart's Clarinet Concerto. It certainly had a profound effect on me: it was as though the music in its very simplicity opened up for a few moments a usually hidden depth to living. The appropriate CD was purchased at the earliest possible opportunity. As a lifelong Methodist I have also of course appreciated moments when a congregation gives one of Wesley's great hymns its best shot and demonstrates that Methodists are still at the top of the league table when it comes to Christian corporate singing.

I have enjoyed a smattering of such experiences over the years. Should they be labelled evidence for the existence of God? Evidence, as sociologist Peter Berger argued in an influential little book some years ago, which might be described as "a rumour of Angels." (2) Certainly they are positive, life enhancing experiences. But was Hans Kung on the right lines for example when he wrote that "to listen to the adagio of the Clarinet Concerto – - – is to perceive something wholly other: the sound of an infinite which transcends and for which "beauty" is no description – - – To describe such experience and revelation of transcendence, religious language still needs the word God." (3)

I am not as persuaded as I once was. I no longer necessarily find a direct link between such experiences and a traditional faith in God. Occasionally I feel like the novelist Julian Barnes: "I don't believe in God but I miss Him." (4) A little more frequently I puzzle over the ambiguities of religion, powerfully captured in these words of another contemporary novelist:

"One person looks around and sees a universe created by a god who watches over its long unfurling, marking the fall of sparrows and listening to the prayers of his finest creation. Another person believes that life, in all its baroque complexity, is a chemical aberration that will briefly decorate the surface of a ball of rock spinning somewhere among 1 billion galaxies. And the two of them could talk for hours and find no great difference between one another for neither set of beliefs make us kinder or wiser. – - – Religion fuelling the turns and reverses of human history, or so it seems, but twist them all to catch a different light and those same passionate beliefs seem no more than banners thrown up to hide the usual engines of greed and fear. And in our single lives? Those smaller turns and reverses? Is it religion which trammels and frees, which gives or withholds hope? Or are these, too, those old base motives dressed up for a Sunday morning? Are they reasons or excuses?" (5)

This is not to surrender to the attack from fundamentalist atheists such as Richard Dawkins. It is to recognise that contemporary insights from biology and physics have posed new forms of the questions with which faith always has to live. Alongside or in the midst of unanswered questions and doubts, I have found that I can empathise with some of the insights of "negative" spirituality or theology which were explored briefly in a previous chapter. No longer chasing after experiences of God which prove to be illusory or indeed non-existent, paradoxically it is the absence of God which most feels like the presence of God. Beyond thought or feeling there is silence, darkness, stillness. There is what Meister Eckhart called "the transcendent abyss" at the heart of us. I want to quote again the lines of RS Thomas which I have already used once: "Why no! I never thought other than / That God is that great absence / In our lives, the empty silence / Within, the place where we go / Seeking, not in hope to / Arrive or find." (6)

Beyond thought and feeling, very aware of the limitations of language, living with unknowable mystery. Whether making use of the image of a dark cloud, a deep abyss or an ocean depth. This mystery is literally incomprehensible. Yet somehow more needs to be said. I guess the key question must be: what might lie at the heart of that darkness, deep within those ocean depths? Inaccessible to rational thought, unknowable, the hunch of faith is that it is not chaos without meaning or a universal indifference. The heart of the darkness, the bedrock at the base of the abyss or the ocean, is love – this is the daring claim at the very centre of Christian faith.

What is the driving force which gives impetus to this leap of faith? The hunch that God is like Jesus! "Although his being is too bright / For human eyes to scan / His meaning lights our shadowed world / Through Christ the Son of Man." (7) The pattern of Jesus – of manger and stable, inclusive ministry, cross and empty tomb – uncovers fundamental truth about human living and indeed the intention behind the whole of creation. It is those truths which convince me and keep me on the path of discipleship. It is that pattern of the life of Christ which is woven together with my life.

The Jewish mystical tradition, according to Rowan Williams, understood that in the creation the presence or glory of God was fragmented, broken into a multitude of separate sparks which could be rediscovered in the lives of the saints. For a Christian, such a spark is seen preeminently in Christ. We glimpse "the light of the knowledge of the glory of God in the face of Jesus Christ." (8) This presence, however, is fundamentally different to what we might have imagined:

"God's Wisdom – - – defines itself in the self forgetting, self emptying love of Christ, the eternal Word, who lives a human life for our sake and is obedient to the point of death. Such Wisdom will always be an exile, a refugee, in a world constrained by endless struggles for advantage, where success lies always in establishing your position at the expense of another's." (9)

So it is that when we use the acclamation at the close of The Lord's Prayer, it is the Kingdom of grace, the power of vulnerability and the glory of self giving love which we are affirming. Although I rather suspect we do not often have those topsy-turvy notions in mind.

"Drained is love in making full; / bound in setting others free; / poor in making many rich; / weak in giving power to be." (10)

To summarise: I live with the absence of God, hidden in a cloud of unknowing. It is being engaged with the endlessly fascinating, demanding and life changing realities of Christ which gives me the courage to believe in creative love rather than meaningless chaos at the heart of things.

In passing, I notice something of a paradox. That although I am very much more aware of the limitations of religious language than I used to be, I still believe in the value of sermons. I think that much of the best preaching has something of the poetic about it, with a careful yet allusive use of words. Moreover, although I have difficulty with prayer which addresses God directly, I still value the cadences of traditional collects and Eucharistic liturgies. It was the Methodist urban theologian John Vincent who once said to me that there was no requirement for theology and spirituality to be logical!

In all this I have found that theology from the perspective of disability is enormously helpful and enlightening. It has provided new insights and raised new questions about how I see Christ and especially the cross and resurrection:

"In the resurrected Jesus Christ (the disciples) saw not the suffering servant for whom the last and most important word was tragedy and sin, but the disabled God who embodied both impaired hands and feet and pierced side, and the imago Dei." (11)

The crucified and risen Lord is seen as the first fruits of new creation. As a Lord who embraces, shares in and affirms the experience of disability, he invites us to ask far reaching questions about how we value different aspects of human living. People with disabilities frequently have less "social capital", they are not achievers in conventional ways. To listen to their varied experiences can result in a subversive undermining of unexamined ideas about status, rewards and the quest for perfection. People with disabilities are no more and no less virtuous than the able-bodied but our very presence challenges any unthinking links between virtue, health and prosperity. Issues around belief in a miracle working interventionist God are given a much sharper focus. Is it more important to see Christ as a miracle worker or as one who shares our infirmities?

For many of my contemporaries, an interest in theology is considered to be rather puzzling if not downright quaint. Yet it has never really occurred to me to give up the enterprise. Indeed I find it difficult to imagine what life would be like without it. From the excitement of new insights to the irritation and raised blood pressure caused by sermons I find bland and superficial – it is all me! I hope, however, that I am not unmindful of some of the awkward questions raised by our context in the 21ˢᵗ-century West. Gordon Lynch outlines some of them:

"Does theology have any useful role to play in helping people think about the meaning of existence, or is it too closely connected to traditional religious ideas to be of any interest or value to the new and emerging ways in which people are pursuing meaning? Can the church have any kind of constructive role in helping the contemporary search for meaning, or will it now be consigned to helping maintain and minister to the religious life of an ever diminishing group of people?" (12)

It was 2004 when increasing disability led me to take the decision to seek early retirement from full-time work. There was much sympathy and kindness within the local Methodist community. Their representatives, working alongside the organisation which provides homes for retired ministers, helped ensure that I ended up in a lovely bungalow well-suited to the needs of a wheelchair user. The process of being awarded an ill-health pension was straightforward. The service to mark my retirement was a moving occasion. Was there anything missing? Yes there was although it has only come properly into focus as I look back. At no point in the process did anyone within the church "system" suggest that we could explore ways in which my active ministry could be continued perhaps on a part-time basis. It seemed as though there was only one choice: between full-time ministry which required certain normative things and retirement. Pastoral ministry requires visiting people in their homes – but most people do not have homes which are wheelchair accessible. Preaching ministry requires conducting two services at least

each Sunday – but I do not have sufficient energy to contem-
plate that level of preaching etc. Administrative ministry
sometimes requires chairing meetings which go on quite late
in the evening – but I have to be home by a certain time to
meet my "put to bed" carers. I think that at the time I was too
traumatised by everything that was happening to be more
proactive myself.

Perhaps my experience throws a little light on a wider issue. Is
the church consistently willing and able to learn from the
insights and make use of the gifts of people with disabilities?
To value their perspectives rather than simply being sympa-
thetic to them? If one part of the renewal of church life
involves listening to and learning from minority groups
(whether in relation to ethnicity, sexuality, gender or disability)
then there is a long way to go. I have found exploring theology
and spirituality from the standpoint of a person with a disability to be exciting and challenging. I do wonder whether the
church as a whole is willing and able to be excited and
challenged by such new voices.

Barbara Glasson writes about the relationship of a variety of
groups to Christian faith and the life of the church including a
group of retired clergy with disabilities. (13) She argues that
the collusion of the church with many of the assumptions
of the wider culture which gives greatest value to "normal"
bodies, competence in work and rational thought actually gets
in the way of the church discovering more of its own true
nature. Owning fragility, vulnerability and struggle as central
aspects of being human is part of the true vocation of the
church as it follows the crucified one. Yet usually the church
values more highly its continuance in the mainstream and
many of its repeated attempts to restructure its organisation,
"to bolster the barricades, to put a new face on old patterns

and to rebrand what has gone before" are driven by that desire. I find much of her trenchant analysis both convincing and challenging.

The several themes that I have tried to explore in these pages live alongside each other. There is the relationship between disability and theology. There are the mountain and desert experiences of stillness, waiting and the absence of God. There is the recognition of the need to pay more attention both to people and things in themselves to discover a little more of the wonder of being alive. There is the continuing conviction that the mysterious relationship between brokenness and blessing which we acknowledge in the Eucharist brings us near to the heart of things. Some notes sound more strongly than others at different times but all are playing. Or, to change the metaphor, all are tributaries flowing into the river which is an ongoing Christian discipleship. I am certainly aware that the relationship between them is far from being moulded into a coherent whole. I hope that they are all making a contribution to that transforming of life and experience which makes Christian living a life long adventure. The search for the true self is not on a bucket list of things to do before I die which can be ticked off. And certainly does not fit into any imagery which suggests that we are always making progress to our final destination. Travelling on the blue highways is much more complex than that. I do rather think though that they give a much deeper encounter with the messy and marvellous realities of life than cruising down the freeway of religious certainty and superiority.

I recognise of course that all this hardly looks like an attractive manifesto for evangelism and making disciples. I confess that I have never knowingly converted anyone. Perhaps there is space within the whole breadth of Christian experience and understanding for the emphases that have come to have a central place for me. Indeed, perhaps they might act as a corrective to very differing perspectives and be corrected themselves in their turn. I hope so.

Meanwhile, I empathise with some words which I think were written by the former Anglican Bishop Richard Holloway: "I wish I had spent less time talking about Jesus and more time following him." If those of us especially who are preachers don't recognise ourselves in those sentiments, then perhaps our true selves have become too well hidden beneath the surface attractions of influence and eloquence which can seduce us.

More widely, I am attracted to Barbara Glasson's suggestions about mission which are rather different from most of what is written. More central to our task than either activity or proclamation, the mission of the church is to stand still so that we become aware that the whole of creation including ourselves is held in God's loving attention. It is in silence that we can become aware of that and from there seek to embody relationships in which we listen both to others and to the natural world. Her suggestion for a sort of mission statement is: "Shut up, keep still and listen!" That seems like a good point at which to end this reflection.

(1) William Least Heat Moon: Blue Highways A Journey into America (Minerva 1993, first published 1983)

(2) Peter Berger: A Rumour of Angels (Pelican 1971)

(3) Hans Kung quoted in Michael Mayne: This Sunrise Of Wonder (1995 new edition Darton, Longman and Todd 2008)

(4) Julian Barnes: Nothing to Be Frightened Of (Vintage 2009)

(5) Mark Haddon: The Red House (Vintage 2013)

(6) RS Thomas: "Via negativa" in Collected Poems 1945-1990 (Phoenix 2000)

(7) Elizabeth Cosnett: "Can we by searching find out God"

(8) II Corinthians 4: 6

(9) Rowan Williams: Christ on Trial (Zondervan 2002)

(10) W H Vanstone: "Morning glory, starlit sky"

(11) Nancy Eiesland: The Disabled God Towards a Liberatory Theology Of Disability (Abingdon Press 1994)

(12) Gordon Lynch: After Religion Generation X and The Search For Meaning (Darton, Longman and Todd 2003)

(13) Barbara Glasson: The Exuberant Church (Darton, Longman and Todd 2011)

IX
Homeward
Bound?

During the period when I was beginning to give some shape to these reflections, my Dad died, on Christmas Day 2013. His had been a long life of over ninety years and a very full life of professional achievement and political and civic service, not to mention more than fifty years as a Methodist local preacher. Typically, he had left meticulous instructions about his funeral service including a recorded rendition of the Welsh national anthem by a male voice choir which we enjoyed both at the crematorium and at the thanksgiving service in church. We also sang lustily that we had strength for today and hope for tomorrow, and that there was no condemnation for us – in relationship with Christ we could approach the eternal throne boldly.

Dad was absolutely convinced that on the far side of death he would be reunited with Mum. That the journey through death would be a homecoming. I am more agnostic, although I have read the words from John 14 (1) about there being many rooms in my Father's house at a hundred funerals. In many a pastoral conversation I have felt the tension between pastoral need and theological hesitation. The former naturally took precedence. Of course you will be reunited with your spouse / parents / siblings / cat / dog.

The theme of exiles and homecomings is a powerful one. It tugs at the heartstrings. Home is "where my love lies waiting silently for me." (2) We rejoice when the sailor comes home from the sea, the soldier returns from the war, the painful and difficult wandering reaches journey's end:

"He said it was the Codex Boturini, about the peregrinations of the Azteca. On the advice of gods they left Aztlan in search of their new home, and took 214 years to find it. The long page was divided into – - – small boxes, each one recording the main thing that happened in that year. – - – Most of the years showed simply their search for home. Anyone could feel the anguish of this book – what longing is keener? Pictographs of weary people walking, carrying babies or weapons. Small, inked footprints trailed down the full length of the book, the sad black tracks of heartache. When completely unfolded, the Codex stretched almost the whole length of the studio. That is how long it is possible to walk, looking for home." (3)

We are pilgrims not strangers. However, we are not so convinced as we once were that the journey is a linear progress towards our eternal home where our immortal souls will find a resting place. Wanting it to be true sits uncomfortably alongside a 21st century scepticism about the likelihood of individual existence extending beyond the grave.

Perhaps the journey is cyclical rather than linear, as some of the poets have suggested. So that "trailing clouds of glory do we come from God who is our home." (4) And eventually "the end of all our exploring will be to arrive where we started and know the place for the first time." (5) We find a phrase, a line, a verse which resonates with us and we wonder whether or not it might be a signpost towards heaven. Yet it seems that Christian focus properly remains on the world that we live in rather than the life of the world to come.

So it is that a much more central question for Christian understanding is how the blue planet can be made more of a home for its inhabitants. One of the more memorable acts of worship I attended took place some forty years ago. It was a Mass for children with a range of physical and intellectual "handicaps" as we called them in those days. The church was packed, with children sitting around the altar and on the steps of the pulpit, and festooned with streamers and balloons. We sang from *Oliver*: "Consider yourself at home, consider yourself one of the family." Incidentally, as the sole Protestant present, I was the only person not permitted to receive Holy Communion.

The Kingdom of God is where people can feel at home: welcomed, valued, affirmed, cherished, forgiven. It is the prodigal son seeing his father come out to meet him on the road and dressing him in the symbols of love and honour. It is the outsiders being welcomed in to share in the banquet. Brian Wren's hymn points to some of its dynamic: justice, joy, challenge, choice, mercy, grace. (6) Discovering ways to feel at home with yourself. Proclaiming, celebrating, joining in that Kingdom work for justice and peace with those who are in one way or another homeless: the dispossessed, the refugees, victims of violence or domestic abuse. More widely still, affirming the need for radical changes in the ways we relate to the planet as a whole. Treating it in ways that affirm it as our common home, not a hotel whose resources we can use without a second thought (although some of my best informed friends on ecological matters have concluded that so much damage has been caused already that it may be too late for it to be reversed).

The image of home is a fruitful one, helping to express several dimensions of Christian good news:

"Basic to our existence is a desire to dwell in a place that welcomes us, an environment worthy of trust and hope, to which we fundamentally belong. We seek the means to inhabit the world and be at home. – - – The basic question of human

109

existence, then, is whether there is welcome at the heart of things. Will I be received and embraced? Is there a voice behind all other voices that says, You are precious, and I will be there for you. Our heart's deepest impulse hankers after connection with a trustworthy creation. – - – In such a place, tragedy is not the final word – hope is." (7)

I believe there is welcome at the heart of things. I am agnostic about whether that will include the continuing beyond death of a personal conscious existence. Perhaps we are like sparks from a bonfire, disappearing into a mysterious darkness in which God is hidden. Or, to change the metaphor, we shall be "plunged in the Godhead's deepest sea / And lost in Thy immensity." (8) And if that should turn out to be an immensity of self giving love which is the heartbeat of the universe? – - – Just a hunch perhaps, but rooted in the mindset of Christ whose story continues to fascinate, inspire and claim me.

(1) John 14: 2

(2) Paul Simon: "Homeward Bound."

(3) Barbara Kingsolver: The Lacuna (Faber and Faber 2010)

(4) William Wordsworth: "Ode, Intimations of Immortality From Recollections Of Early Childhood."

(5) TS Eliot: "Little Gidding" in Collected Poems 1909-1962 (Faber and Faber 1963)

(6) Brian Wren: "The kingdom of God is justice and joy."

(7) Thomas Reynolds: Vulnerable Communion A Theology Of Disability and Hospitality (Brazos Press, 2008)

(8) Charles Wesley: "Come, Holy Ghost, all-quickening fire"

Lightning Source UK Ltd.
Milton Keynes UK
UKOW02f1225121115

262526UK00002B/31/P

9 781781 489758